Amel Ben hamad
Nadia Kolsi
Mahdi Ben Dhaou

Urinary tract infection in newborns

Amel Ben hamad
Nadia Kolsi
Mahdi Ben Dhaou

Urinary tract infection in newborns

clinical, diagnostic, treatment, prevention

ScienciaScripts

Imprint

Cover image: www.ingimage.com

This book is a translation from the original published under ISBN 978-620-6-72599-2.

Publisher:
Sciencia Scripts
is a trademark of
Dodo Books Indian Ocean Ltd. and OmniScriptum S.R.L publishing group

120 High Road, East Finchley, London, N2 9ED, United Kingdom
Str. Armeneasca 28/1, office 1, Chisinau MD-2012, Republic of Moldova, Europe
Printed at: see last page
ISBN: 978-620-8-25567-1

Table of contents

INTRODUCTION

Neonatal urinary tract infection is one of the most worrying pathologies in neonatology, due to its frequency and potential severity.

It affects 0.1 to 1% of full-term births and 4 to 25% of premature births, with a clear male predominance. Diagnosis is based on leukocyturia >=10/mm3 and bacteriuria >=10^5 CFU/ml. Considerable progress has been made in the management of neonatal urinary tract infection, but there is as yet no clear consensus on how it should be managed. Its severity is due to the immaturity of the newborn's immune defenses. The most serious long-term complications are arterial hypertension in 26% of cases, and renal failure in 10%.

Neonatal urinary tract infection has not received much attention in the literature, despite its peculiarities at neonatal age, namely:

- Clinical symptoms are unspecific, with urinary signs virtually absent in most cases.
- Rapid progression to sepsis
- Frequent association with malformative uropathies justifying systematic radiological explorations from the 1er episode.
- Difficulty of sterile urine collection (incontinent population)
- Treatment must be urgent, with systematic hospitalization and initiation of intravenous dual therapy. The aim of the treatment is to sterilize the urine and prevent the appearance of kidney scars on an immature kidney whose nephron multiplication is very active.

EPIDEMIOLOGY

1. EPIDEMIOLOGICAL ASPECTS OF NEONATAL URINARY TRACT INFECTIONS :

1.1. Frequency :

Urinary tract infection is relatively common in the neonatal period. It affects 0.1 to 1% of full-term births and 4 to 25% of premature births (1).

In neonatal wards, the frequency of UTIs is estimated at between 7.5 and 15% in neonates hospitalized in intensive care units (2), and between 0.15 and 5.5% in all hospitalized neonates (3,4).

1.2. Breakdown by gender :

Male predominance is found in the literature, with a sex ratio ranging from 1.8 to 9 (Table I). This predominance could be explained by the presence of phimosis, the frequency of uropathy and the susceptibility of males to infection (1).

In infants over 3 months of age and older children, UTIs are much more common in girls (5,6). The prevalence of UTIs in boys over 1 year of age is estimated at less than 0.2%, while it is over 1% in girls of the same age, and as high as 3.5%. (7)

Table I: Comparison of sex ratios in newborns with UTIs in different studies

Author's name	Year	Sex ratio (M/F)
Youssef (2)	2012	1.8
Bergstrom (8)	1972	2,8
Atmani (3)	2007	4,7
Lopez (1)	2007	5,3
Gérard (4)	1998	9

1.3. Age distribution :

Urine culture should not be part of the traditional evaluation of sepsis in the first 72 hours of life. Neonates under 72 hours of age do not acquire UTIs, probably because of the low glomerular filtration rate, the low concentrating capacity of urine or the ability to disrupt bacterial adhesion to the urinary epithelium at this age (9,10).

In the study by Atmani et al, the mean age of onset of symptomatology was 9 days, with a mean age on admission of 14 days; in the study by Gérard et al, the mean age of onset of symptomatology was 11.4 days, with a mean age on admission of 14 days; and in the study by Lopez et al, the mean age on admission was 16 days (1,3,4).

CLINIC

1. CLINICAL ASPECTS OF URINARY TRACT INFECTION IN NEWBORNS :

Neonatal urinary tract infections (UTIs) are characterized by their heterogeneous, non-specific and often misleading clinical symptoms, and their frequent progression to sepsis(4,11-13).

In adults and older children, urinary signs are in the 1er foreground, unlike in newborns, in whom urinary signs may be absent (14).

The risk of sepsis varies from 4% to 7% in full-term newborns and from 10% to 14% in premature infants, which is rare in adults (15-17).

1.1. Thermal disturbance :

As in infants and older children, fever is a common sign of neonatal UTIs (4,18,19). In many cases, it is the only initial symptom(20).

In the literature, the diagnosis of UTI was made in 46% of cases in the Nejjari series (21), in 16% of cases in the Gérard series (4) and in 15% of cases in the Oukkadi series (22).

Thus, urinary tract infection should be considered in the presence of any unexplained febrile state in the neonatal period (20).

However, fever is not constant. It may be absent in around 50% of cases, or may even be replaced by hypothermia. Its absence does not exclude the diagnosis of UTI in newborns (4,5,23).

1.2. Digestive signs:

Digestive signs may include diarrhea, vomiting, abdominal distension, feeding difficulties and hepatosplenomegaly. They are common in neonatal UTIs (Table II).

They may be in the 1er foreground, with no associated thermal imbalance, and can therefore lead to delayed diagnosis and management (24).

Table II: Comparison of the frequency of digestive signs during neonatal urinary tract infection in different studies

Author's name	Digestive signs	Diarrhea	Vomiting	Abdominal bloating	HMG	SMG	Refusal to feed
Gérard (4)	37	12	25	4	25	2	-
Sayah(25)	20	11,3	9,7	6,4	8,1	3,2	16,3
Oukaddi (22)	59,2	18,5	27,8	12,9	9,25	3,9	33,3
Hallab (26)	49,8	19,1	22,7	8	5,5	-	39,3

1.3. Weight anomalies :

In the absence of any intake deficiency or dietary intolerance, weight abnormalities (loss, stagnation or poor weight gain) are highly suggestive of urinary tract infection in newborns, testifying to a process evolving over several days or even weeks (4,8,18,27).

Their frequency varies from study to study, at around 6% in the series by Sayeh and Soufi (21,25); 43% in the series by Bergstrom (8); 61.1% in the series by Oukkadi (22) and 79% in the series by Gérard (4).

1.4. Jaundice:

The frequency of jaundice in UTIs varies from 6% to 26% in the various studies. It is estimated at 6% in Gérard's study (4); 9.25% in Oukkadi's study (22); 16.3% in Sayeh's study (25) and 26% in Hallab's study (26).

Other studies have evaluated the frequency of urinary tract infection in newborns with unexplained jaundice. In the study by Bilgen et al. of 102 newborns born with unexplained jaundice in the first two weeks of life, 8% developed a urinary tract infection (28). In the study by Xinias et al. the rate of urinary tract infection was estimated at 6.5% in newborns aged 3 to 25 days with unexplained jaundice (29).

Although the pathophysiological relationship between hyperbilirubinemia and urinary tract infections remains poorly elucidated, several authors have suspected a dual etiopathogenesis: hemolytic (oxidative stress-induced acceleration of heme-to-bilirubin conversion) and retentional (direct invasion of the liver by bacteria disseminated by the blood or lymphatic route, aggression of the liver by bacterial toxins, or cellular anoxia, fever-related damage, undernutrition) (30-32).

Thus, in the presence of any unexplained prolonged jaundice in a newborn, whether febrile or not, it is imperative to perform an ECBU in search of a urinary tract infection (32).

1.5. Urinary manifestations:

Although urinary signs are less frequent in the neonatal period, questioning may reveal haematuria, pyuria, cloudy urine, abnormalities of the urinary stream such as drip micturition, or incessant crying during micturition (4,13). A review of the literature shows that the frequency of urinary signs varies from 1.2% to 16.7% in different studies (4,21,22,26).

1.6. Neurological manifestations:

Neurological signs such as lethargy, irritability, hypotonia and hyporeactivity may be present, but are not specific to UTI. The presence of these signs should prompt an imperative search for associated bacterial meningitis (33,34).

1.7. Sepsis :

Urinary tract infection is frequently complicated by sepsis (35), but rarely leads to septic shock (4,27).

In Bauer's study, urinary tract infections were diagnosed during sepsis assessments, which included blood count, blood cultures, urine cytobacteriological examination and lumbar puncture. Urine cultures were only taken in septic assessments performed after 72 h (35).

For this reason, ECBU should be part of the systematic work-up for sepsis from D3 onwards.

Moreover, the hematogenous origin of urinary tract infection is very common at this age. As a result, other secondary localizations are possible: meningeal, articular and hepatic (36).

BACTERIOLOGY

1. BACTERIOLOGICAL DIAGNOSIS :

The doctor's role is to rigorously describe the steps required to guarantee quality data collection (37).

1.1. Local disinfection :

Disinfection is essential before any urine sample is taken, to ensure maximum sterility.

Disinfection of the periurethral area is performed with chlorhexidine or soap, followed by rinsing with sterile water or saline to prevent any antiseptic from passing into the urine. For female newborns, it is performed from front to back, and for uncircumcised male newborns, it is performed after decapping (5,38).

1.2. Sampling methods :

Urine must be collected sterile and cultured immediately, whatever the method of collection. If urine cannot be inoculated quickly, it can be stored at 4°C for 24 hours (39).

There are several methods of urine collection:

1.2.1. Urine collection using a collection bag:

The collection bag is the easiest and most widely used method for newborns, as they are unable to urinate voluntarily. To minimize the risk of contamination, the external genitalia must be thoroughly disinfected, and the bag should not be left in place for more than 30 minutes.

Studies have shown that the average collection time is estimated at 40 min, with a maximum of 4 hours. Therefore, if the newborn does not urinate after 30 minutes, the bag must be changed, and local disinfection is required before inserting the new bag (37,40).

If urine stagnates in the bag, there will be no change in the leukocyte count, but rather bacterial proliferation will be enhanced. The reliability of this technique can reach 85% for a single sample, and even 95% for two successive samples. (41).

The American Academy of Pediatrics (AAP) guidelines state that urine cultures collected by bag have an unacceptable false-positive rate of 88-99%, and are only valid when they give negative results. To establish a reliable diagnosis of UTI in non-continental patients, they recommend that the sample should be obtained by catheterization or suprapubic puncture (42).

Although actively discouraged by the AAP, urine collection by adhesive bag remains an easy method, widely used in France, particularly in emergency departments (40,42).

This is the preferred mode of collection in Europe: out of 1129 paediatricians surveyed, 53% chose the bag as their first choice for infants < 3 months and 59% for children aged 4 to 36 months (43) , while in the USA, 25% of samples from 3066 infants were collected by bag, 70% by catheter, 3% by catheterization and 2% by self-administration (44).

1.2.2. Urine collection with a pad :

This collection method involves disinfecting the perineum, followed by inserting the pad into the newborn's diaper. Trapped urine is then aspirated from the pad after micturition.

There are pads designed for this purpose, such as the Newcastle urine collection pad, but this product is unavailable in Tunisia. (Figure 21)

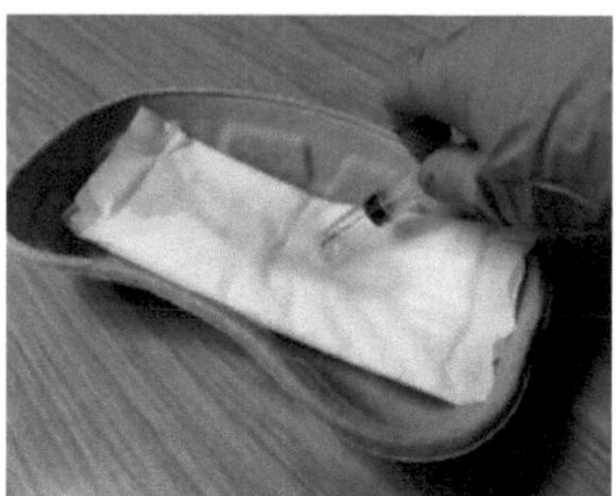

Figure 1: Urine collection pad

The likelihood of missing urine is greatly reduced when using tampons, with a sampling success rate of around 96%. Parents prefer this method, as it requires less parental effort and causes little disturbance to their child (45,46).

Urine collection swabs trap a significant amount of cellular material, reducing the number of cells available for microscopy, but strip tests for blood and leukocyte esterase remain reliable (47-50).

Contamination by skin or intestinal flora is the main concern when using urine collection pads, due to the prolonged contact between the pad and the perineum. To reduce this risk, measures such as the use of moisture-sensitive alarms and changing the pad every 30 minutes were tested. Alarms did not prove effective in reducing contamination. Changing the pad every 30 min, evaluated in a randomized controlled trial, resulted in a contamination rate of 3%, compared with 29% when a single pad was left in place (41,51).

Comparing urine collection with tampons and collection with a jet, we found that the probability of sample contamination was significantly increased, and that the prevalence of urinary tract infections was lower with tampons.

Indeed, the contamination rate varies from 12.2% to 26.3% for tampons versus 1.8% to 6.4% for squirts, and the prevalence of UTIs is estimated at 1.3% for tampons versus 2.3% for squirts, suggesting that UTIs are missed in samples collected by tampons due to contamination (52,53).

The presence of squamous epithelial cells on microscopy is predictive of contamination in urine collected in the jet. It indicates the passage of urine over the skin. On the other hand, for urine collected through tampons, the presence or absence of squamous cells should not be taken into consideration, as there is prolonged contact of the tampons with the skin (53).

1.2.3. Jet urine collection :

This technique can be used at any age, but is much easier to perform in older children (45). The DUTY study carried out in the UK showed that the method of collection varies according to age: for children under 3 years of age, 26.3% of samples were collected by squirting, compared with 96.7% for children aged 3 to 5 years (52).

Initially, the newborn is prepared by feeding at the breast or with a bottle to fill the bladder. After 25 minutes, the perineum is cleansed and a sterile container is held under the urethra to collect the urine (Figure 22). Care should be taken to avoid skin contact with the sample container (21,42,54).

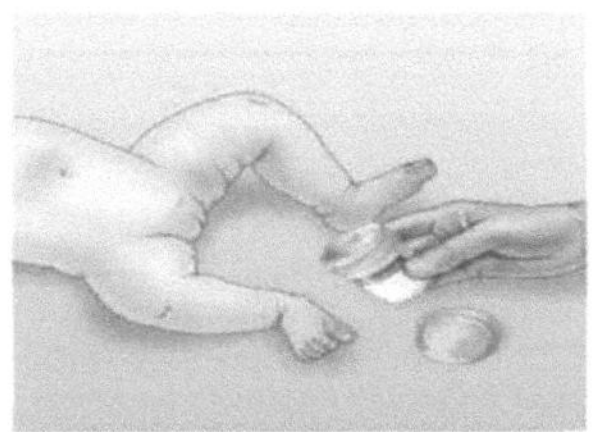

Figure 2: Urine stream collection

Contamination rates vary considerably between studies (Table III).

Table III: Comparison of the contamination rate of urine collected in the urine stream in the different studies

The study	The year	Contamination rate (%)
Macfarlane et al (55)	1999	27
Alam et al (45)	2005	14,7
Tosif et al (56)	2012	26
Ho et al (57)	2014	4,5
Teo et al (58)	2016	16-38

Jet urine collection can be time-consuming, with a median sampling time of 30.5 min. urine is missed in around 16% of attempts. A combination of these factors may contribute to collection failure, leading to abandonment of this method in 20% of cases (59).

1.2.4. Stimulation of urination :

Non-invasive tests rely on the child's spontaneous urination. Stimulating urination could shorten urine collection time, leaving less time for contamination to occur.

In neonates, central inhibition of spinal reflex arcs is less developed. Micturition can be stimulated in the following way, using the method of Herreros et al: The baby is held upright under both armpits with legs dangling. The suprapubic abdomen is tapped at 100 taps/min for 30 s, alternating with a circular lumbosacral massage for 30 s, for a duration of 5 min (Figure 23).

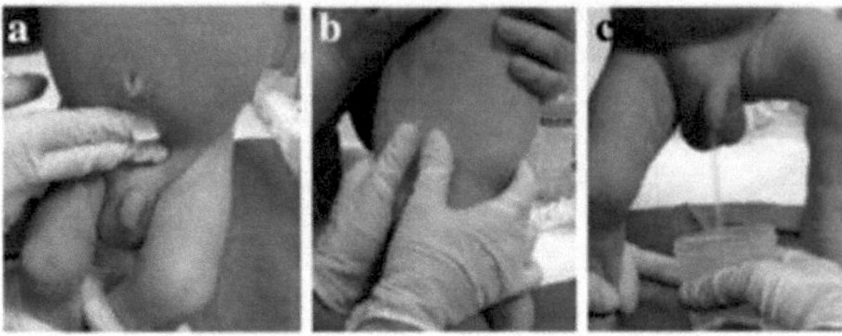

a) Tapoter l'abdomen sus-pubien b) Massage lombosacré circulaire
c) Collection des urines au jet par un flacon stérile

Figure 3: Stimulation of micturition using the technique of Herreros et al.

This maneuver has been shown to promote micturition, particularly if performed 30 minutes after feeding (60). Use of this technique in neonates less than 7 days old resulted in micturition within 5 minutes in 90% of cases (61).

Applying this technique to a population with an average age of 6 to 7 days, micturition was obtained in 86.3% of cases, with an estimated median collection time of 45 s (60). In direct comparison with neonates aged less than 10 days, 78% of stimulated neonates urinated within 5 min, compared with 33% of unstimulated controls (54).

The effectiveness of the technique decreases with age. For infants under 6 months, stimulation led to micturition in 49% of cases, with a median collection time of 45 seconds (62).

A study by Valleix et al, revealed a success rate of 27% in a population of infants with a median age of 10 months, with a collection time of 2 minutes in the majority of successful attempts (63). This probability of success decreased with increasing infant weight (63).

Another method of voiding stimulation has been studied: the

"Quick-Wee" technique by Kaufman et al (Figure 24).

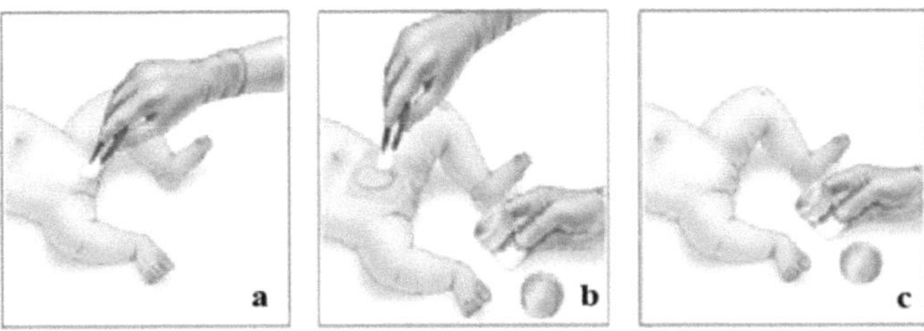

a) Désinfection b) Mouvements circulaires en sus-pubien
c) Collection des urines au jet par un flacon stérile

Figure 4: Stimulation of micturition using the "Quick Wee" method

The first step involves peri-genital cleansing at room temperature. The second step consists in using a sterile compress cooled to 2.8°C, soaked in physiological saline and held in place by disposable plastic forceps, to make continuous circular movements until micturition is obtained or 5 minutes of stimulation are reached.

In infants aged 1 to 12 months, stimulated for up to 5 minutes, micturition was obtained in 31% of cases versus 12% of unstimulated controls (64). (64)No difference was reported in the contamination rate, estimated at 27%, which is similar to other studies of jet-collected samples (64). The use of ultrasound to determine bladder fullness prior to stimulation did not alter the success rate of the technique within 5 minutes (65).

1.2.5. Suprapubic bladder puncture:

Suprapubic vesical puncture is often described as the gold standard for urine collection. It is the only method that allows the urethra to be short-circuited, thus avoiding contamination by bacteria that colonize the distal urethra (42,66).

However, suprapubic puncture is also considered the most invasive and painful method by doctors and parents (67). Indeed, this technique can be complicated by transient microscopic hematuria (3.6%), especially in hypotrophic children, macroscopic hematuria (1%), abdominal wall abscesses, intestinal perforation (0.71%) or bacteremia (42,68).

In a contemporary evaluation by parents and nurses of newborns and infants under 60 days of age, puncture was judged more painful than catheterization (68).

The abdominal location of the full bladder in the neonatal period facilitates the use of this technique in this age group. After 1 hour or more since the last micturition, the skin is disinfected and the bladder is punctured with a small catheter inclined at 20° to 30° to the vertical, at the midline, 1 cm above the pubic symphysis. Aspirate until a few millilitres of urine are obtained, then remove the catheter. The puncture site should be compressed (69). (Figure 25)

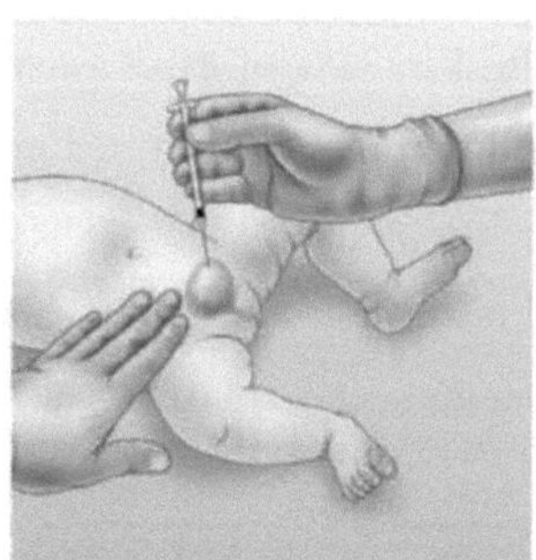

Figure 5: Suprapubic puncture

An ultrasound-guided approach gave good results in infants and older children, but showed no significant benefit in neonates, with an estimated success rate of 74% for unguided punctures versus 75% for guided punctures (42).

Bacterial growth on urine collected by suprapubic puncture may be considered a urinary tract infection, given the low risk of contamination (70). However, some centers require a lower culture threshold than those applied to other sampling methods.

The thresholds recommended by the Italian Society of Pediatric Nephrology (SINP): 1 × 104 cfu/ml from puncture or catheterized samples, 5 × 104 cfu/ml from jet samples and 1 × 105 cfu/ml from bag samples (71).

The American Academy of Pediatrics suggests combining leukocyturia with a bacteriuria threshold of 5 × 104 cfu/ml to retain UTI regardless of collection method in children under 2 years of age, in order to eliminate contamination (72).

1.2.6. Bladder catheterization :

This method involves inserting a bladder catheter until a few drops of urine are obtained, then removing the catheter. Urine collection by bladder catheterization avoids contamination by bacteria that colonize the distal urethra. Ideally, the first few drops of urine should be discarded, as they are more likely to be contaminated by urethral bacteria. Indeed, a randomized comparison of early and late sampling revealed greater contamination for the sample containing the first drops (73).

The contamination rate ranged from 1% to 28.6% in the various studies, indicating better performance than other non-invasive methods (54,56,58,74,75). However, a study by Herreros et al. in 60 infants under 90 days of age, compared jet and catheter samples from the same patient, showing a contamination rate of 5% for jet urine versus 8% for catheter urine (76).

Although this technique is effective, its use should be avoided as far as possible in children, particularly newborns, as it is painful, causes urethral trauma, particularly in boys, and can be complicated by sepsis (66).

The National Institute for Health and Clinical Excellence (NICE) recommends jet urine collection as the 1st-line method. If jet collection is not possible, it recommends other non-invasive methods as a second-line option. Bladder catheterization and suprapubic puncture are considered to be the most accurate sampling methods from a diagnostic point of view, but are only recommended as a third-line method because of their invasive nature (77).

The American Academy of Pediatrics (AAP) requires urine collection by catheterization or puncture to establish the diagnosis of UTI, if antibiotics are to be administered (72).

1.3. Urine transport and storage:

Germs can multiply in urine at room temperature. Certain precautions must therefore be taken when transporting and storing urine.

The expert panel of the American Society for Microbiology and the Infectious Diseases Society of America agreed that urine should not be left at room temperature for more than 30 minutes. It should be kept refrigerated (2°C to 10°C) if not cultured within 30 minutes of collection. (78)

NICE recommends that urine should not be left at room temperature for longer than 4 hours. If urine cannot be cultured within 4 hours of collection, it should be stored immediately in the refrigerator, or using a bacteriostatic agent (boric acid).

The manufacturer's instructions should also be followed when using boric acid, to ensure that the sample volume is correct and thus avoid any potential toxicity to the bacteria present in the sample (79).

Refrigeration should not exceed 24 hours, and does not prevent cell lysis. Bacteria can therefore be counted reliably, while leukocytes may be altered from the 12ème hour mark. Boric acid enables urine to be stored at room temperature for 48 hours, without significantly altering bacteriuria and leukocyturia (37).

1.4. Cytobacteriological examination of urine:

1.4.1. Macroscopic examination :

It essentially provides information on the color and appearance of the urine. This examination is of little interest. Cloudy urine does not necessarily mean infection. Turbidity may be due to the presence of crystals. And clear urine is not always sterile. In 5% of cases, it may conceal an infection. What's more, urine discoloration does not indicate the presence of hematuria, which can be caused by medication such as rifampicin (37).

1.4.2. Direct microscopic examination :

Direct examination should be carried out as soon as the urine arrives at the laboratory, so that results can be communicated as quickly as possible. It enables both cytological and bacteriological studies to be carried out(66).

1.4.2.1. Cytological examination :

Cytological examination identifies and quantifies leukocytes, red blood cells and cylinders. It can also reveal the presence of crystals and epithelial cells.

Leukocyturia of less than 10/mm3 or 10,000/ml corresponds to renal filtration of leukocytes (66).

Significant leukocyturia, greater than 10/mm3 or 10,000/ml, indicates the presence of an inflammatory process in the urinary tract (37).

Significant leukocyturia strongly suggests urinary tract infection. However, it is not pathognomonic.

There are situations in which a UTI can be found without leukocyturia, such as prior antibiotic therapy, alkaline urine pH, long storage of urine in the refrigerator, delayed inflammatory reaction, urine collected at an early stage of UTI (38,66).

There are other situations in which leukocyturia can be found without urinary infection, such as in the case of concentrated urine found especially in dehydrated subjects, irritation by urinary catheterization, or the presence of kidney stones (66).

1.4.2.2. Bacteriological examination :

Bacteriological examination provides information on the presence of bacteria, their morphology, grouping, mobility and response to Gram staining.

The definition of bacteriuria is based on the presence of bacteria in the urine. This bacteriuria may indicate contamination or a true urinary tract infection(80).

Although quantitative bacteriuria is more reliable than direct examination for germs, the latter can be very useful. Its results are best obtained on centrifuged urine.

A positive direct examination on stained centrifuged urine indicates bacteriuria greater than 5x104 CFU/ml. Its sensitivity on centrifuged urine varies from 60% to 100%, and its specificity from 59% to 97% in various studies (66).

Given the sterility of urine and the possibility of contamination by faecal or genital flora, interpretation at the end of direct examination must take into account clinical symptomatology, the number and nature of species present, and concomitant abnormalities on cytological examination, in order to guide the neonatologist in the choice of treatment (37,80).

1.4.3. Urine culture :

1.4.3.1. Germ count :

Urine culture is performed on selective media. The germ responsible for the urinary tract infection is isolated, counted and tested for antibiotic sensitivity. Results are available after 24 to 48 hours of incubation. (80)

The interpretation of this count is based on the Kass criteria:

For urine collected in a stream,

- In case of bacteriuria greater than or equal to 10^5 germs/ml with a single species isolated ⅜ Confirmed infection
- In case of bacteriuria less than or equal to 10^3 germs/ml ⅜ Infection invalidated (exception: the case of the newborn under antibiotic treatment with a monomicrobial culture less than or equal to 10^3 germs/ml).
- In case of bacteriuria between 10^3 and 10^5 germs/ml: This may be an early infection, an infection masked by the antibiotic or simply very dilute urine ⅜ repeat the examination

According to Kass, the significant threshold for bacteriuria is 10^4 germs/ml for urine collected by bladder catheterization, and 10^2 germs/ml for urine collected by suprapubic puncture (5).

The Kass criteria made the exception for the case of the newborn under antibiotic treatment with a monomicrobial culture less than or equal to 10^3 germs/ml, but they did not take into consideration a frequent situation: the presence of significant leukocyturia without bacteriuria, which in most cases testifies to a non-infectious inflammatory process, but which may reflect a urinary tract infection decapitated by antibiotic therapy (37).

1.4.3.2. Germs involved :

A review of the literature reveals that the germs most frequently encountered in neonatal UTIs are Enterobacteriaceae. *E.coli* is the predominant germ in all reported series. Its frequency ranges from 48% to 81%. *Kpneumoniae* comes next in the majority of studies, with a frequency ranging from 5.3% to 21.4% (4,8,21).

1.4.3.3. Antibiotic susceptibility testing :

Antibiotic susceptibility testing for urinary tract infections should be performed systematically, especially when resistant strains are emerging. The reading takes 24 hours. The aim is to adapt antibiotic treatment.

Antibiograms are used to study the action of antibiotics on bacterial growth in vitro.

The disc method is the most widely used. It studies only the bacteriostatic action of the antibiotic tested, by determining the minimum inhibitory concentration (MIC). This MIC is then compared with the antibiotic's blood concentration (APC) obtained with the usual dosage:

- The strain is said to be sensitive if the MIC is lower than the CSA.
- The strain is said to be intermediate if the MIC is close to the CSA.
- The strain is said to be resistant if the MIC is greater than the CSA.

In our series, all newborns had undergone antibiotic susceptibility testing.

Maximum sensitivity was noted for imipenem (97.73%), followed by amikacin (88.64%) and gentamicin (75%), in line with the literature.

Overall sensitivity to cefotaxime was 70.45%.

1.5. The role of urine dipsticks in diagnosis :

The diagnosis of urinary tract infection is suspected clinically, based on a number of factors confirmed by ECBU.

Reactivate strips are widely used to detect urinary tract infections in adults and older children. They are used to test for leukocyte esterase and nitrite.

Urine must be fresh and have been in the bladder for more than 3 hours.

Strip reading times vary according to the test: leukocyte testing requires 2 minutes, while 30 seconds is sufficient for the detection of nitrate reductase activity in enterobacteria (37,38).

Leukocyte esterase (LE) is an enzyme produced by white blood cells. It is found in urine where white blood cells have been active, as in the case of urinary tract infection. A high false-negative rate is noted in neutropenic patients and in neonates and very young infants, due to frequent urination, which reduces the accumulation of LE in stored urine.

Nitrite is the product of the reduction of dietary nitrate to nitrite. This takes place via enterobacteria with nitrate reductase activity (37,38,42).

Thus, in newborns and very young infants, strips are not a reliable means of screening for urinary tract infection for several reasons:

- Frequent urination
- Low-nitrate milk diet
- Physiological leukocyturia may occur in the first few days
- Possible infection by germs that do not reduce nitrates to nitrites (42)

BIOLOGY

1. BIOLOGICAL MARKERS OF URINARY TRACT INFECTION

:

Biomarkers are used for several purposes:

- Positive diagnosis and diagnosis of severity of infection
- Monitoring treatment progress
- Prediction of possible renal sequelae

The most commonly used markers are : C-reactive protein, procalcitonin and interleukins 6 and 8 (81).

1.1. C-reactive protein (CRP):

C-reactive protein (CRP) is a protein of the acute phase of inflammation, secreted by liver cells between 4 and 6 hours after the onset of infection, reaching a peak between 36 and 48 hours. (82,83).

CRP is the marker most commonly available in hospitals. It is a validated marker, used both to diagnose bacterial infection and to monitor progress under treatment. (81,84)

Given its kinetics, CRP is not a good means of early diagnosis, but it has been shown that infection can be excluded if a 2ème CRP assay after 24 hours of suspicion is negative (81).

CRP falls rapidly with antibiotic treatment of the germ responsible for the infection. However, it remains elevated in the event of ineffective treatment. Thus, CRP is predictive of antibiotic efficacy (84,85).

CRP lacks specificity for bacterial infections. Its level may increase considerably in patients with viral infections, malignant tumors, severe trauma and autoimmune diseases(86,87).

In reviewing the literature, some authors had suggested a correlation between elevated CRP values and the occurrence of renal scarring, but this correlation was not subsequently validated (84,88).

1.2. Procalcitonin (PCT):

During the first two days of life, PCT can be physiologically increased up to 21 pg/l. Consequently, special reference values must be used for premature babies and neonates under 48 hours of age. From the 3rd day of life, the reference values are those used for adults, detailed as follows:

Rate interpretation :

- If PCT level < 0.5 μg/l, bacterial origin can be ruled out except in cases of strong clinical suspicion, when PCT must be re-dosed 12 to 24 hours after the 1st assay.
- If PCT levels are between 0.5 and 2 μg/l, the diagnosis is not certain.

  The MDT must be re-dosed 24 hours later.
- If PCT levels > 2 pg/l, bacterial infection is highly probable
- If PCT > 10 pg/l, the diagnosis of septic shock is almost certain. (89,90)

PCT kinetics :

During a bacterial infection, PCT secretion begins between 2 and 6 hours, peaking between 12 and 16 hours (82).

PCT can help in the early diagnosis of neonatal bacterial infections and in differentiating between viral and bacterial infection. Studies have shown that serum procalcitonin has better sensitivity and specificity than CRP in terms of early diagnosis of neonatal sepsis, diagnosis of severity of infection and in assessing response to antibiotic treatment (87,91).

In terms of urinary tract infection, the severity of renal damage correlates with high serum procalcitonin concentrations (92).

1.3. Cytokines: interleukin 6 (IL-6) and 8 (IL-8) :

Interleukins 6 and 8 are markers of severe bacterial infection. They are not specific for urinary tract infection.

IL-6 is a multifunctional cytokine: it is a pyrogenic substance involved in hematopoiesis, in the production of inflammation proteins in the acute phase, it activates lymphocytes and increases immunoglobulin A secretion. Several cells synthesize this cytokine, namely macrophages, fibroblasts, cellular endothelial cells and renal tubular epithelial cells (93).

IL-8 is a chemokine characterized by its chemotactic effect on neutrophils. It is produced mainly by activated monocytes, endothelial cells, keratinocytes and fibroblasts. Production is induced by lipopolysaccharides, tumor necrosis factor (TNF-α), IL-1 and IL-2. Mesangial cells and cortical epithelia of the kidney also express and secrete IL-8 (94,95).

IL-6 and IL-8 are important cytokines produced in response to severe neonatal bacterial infections such as sepsis, meningitis and urinary tract infection (96).

A study by Roilides et al (96) of 27 neonates with urinary tract infections measured blood and urine concentrations of IL-6 and IL-8 at the start of the infection and at the second week of treatment, and performed dimercapto-succinic acid-technetium-99m (DMSA) scans between 10 and 90 days after the urinary tract infection.

Increased concentrations of IL-6 and IL-8 were observed in urine, but not in serum within 24 hours of the presumed diagnosis of UTI, testifying to the production of inflammatory cytokines by the neonatal urinary tract in response to uropathogens.

All neonates showed undetectable levels of urinary cytokines during the second week of treatment.

DMSA scans showed pyelonephric changes in 15 neonates (56%).

These renal alterations on scans correlate with elevated urinary IL-6 concentrations, but with no significant correlation to IL-8 concentrations.

Thus, IL-6 can serve as a predictive marker for renal sequelae.

However, these assays are not widely used due to their high cost.

RADIOLOGY

1. RADIOLOGICAL INVESTIGATION OF URINARY TRACT INFECTION :

Imaging has no place in the diagnosis of urinary tract infection in neonates. It is useful for diagnosing complications and highlighting underlying urological abnormalities (97).

1.1. Renal ultrasound:

Renal ultrasound is the 1st-line examination for the investigation of urinary tract infection in newborns. It is a non-invasive, non-irradiating and accessible examination that enables morphological and structural analysis of the urinary tract:

- The kidney: number and position, contours, biometry (cortical thickness, dimensions of pyelocalic cavities, measurement of the anteroposterior diameter of the pyelon), cortico-medullary differentiation.
- The ureters: not visible in the normal state
- Bladder: size, wall thickness and appearance, echogenicity (98).

In line with NICE recommendations in Switzerland and the UK, all newborns with a urinary tract infection should undergo renal ultrasound. Ultrasound should be performed at a distance from the infection, to ensure more accurate interpretation of the urinary tract. Indeed, if performed early, it can detect transient abnormalities of the renal parenchyma caused by tissue edema, or dilatation of the pyelocalic cavities induced by bacterial endotoxins. But in the event of sepsis, bladder globe, impaired diuresis or renal function, or lack of improvement after 48 hours of treatment, it should be performed during the acute phase (48-72 h) to detect possible infectious complications such as renal abscess, perirenal abscess, pyonephrosis, etc., or obstructive uropathy. (72,79,99)

1.2. Retrograde urethrocystography (RUC):

UCR is the method of choice for diagnosing vesicoureteral reflux. It is an invasive, radiating and costly examination which allows accurate classification of VUR, identification of posterior urethral valves and bladder and ureteral anomalies (98). Vesico-ureteral reflux may be intermittent and subsequently may not be visualized on UCR. Thus, a normal UCR does not rule out the presence of VUR (100).

Based on Swiss and British NICE recommendations, UCR is indicated in newborns in cases of atypical urinary tract infection, recurrent urinary tract infection, ultrasound abnormalities or a family history of vesico-ureteral reflux. A urinary tract infection is said to be atypical if there are hemodynamic disorders, a bladder globe, if there is an impact on diuresis or renal function, or if there is no improvement after 48 hours of treatment. It is said to be recurrent if it recurs at least once (79,99).

UCR should be performed after urine sterilization, due to the risk of infection (24). Several studies have attempted to determine the optimum time between infection and the performance of UCR: some authors have supported the idea of performing UCR within 3 to 6 weeks, as the infection may cause transient reflux, but Craig et al, Mac Donald et al and Sanjay et al have shown that the results of UCR performed during the first week of UTI are not influenced. They have also shown that performing UCR in the acute phase has several benefits:

- Reduce the number of people lost without exploration
- Enable rapid planning of management strategies
- Minimize the need for antibiotic prophylaxis while waiting for the

UCR, thereby reducing the rate of bacterial resistance (101-104).

According to the recommendations of the Swiss Pediatric Society, once UCR has been indicated, it should be performed as soon as possible, under antibiotic prophylaxis if the newborn or infant is not on antibiotic treatment (99).

1.3. Renal scintigraphy :

Scintigraphy is a non-invasive, low-radiation examination for morpho-functional analysis of the urinary tract. The two most commonly used tracers are dimercapto-succinic acid-technétium 99m (DMSA) and mercapto-acetyl-triglycine-technétium 99m (MAG3) (39,105).

1.3.1. DMSA scintigraphy:

DMSA is a static tracer characterized by its affinity for the renal cortex and its poor excretion. Because of its slow renal uptake, analysis of images taken 2 to 6 hours after administration enables :

- Diagnosing acute pyelonephritis
- Look for kidney scars
- Quantifying renal function (105)

Its use in the acute phase is increasingly rare (11). After an infectious episode lasting 4 to 6 months, it is indicated in cases of atypical or recurrent urinary tract infection, or in cases of ultrasound anomalies (11,98,106).

The European Society of Urology recommends two approaches to the diagnosis of RVU (107):

- The bottom-up approach, which consists of performing a UCR and then completing with a DMSA scan if cystography is positive.
- Top-down approach: DMSA scan followed by UCR if scan is

positive

1.3.2. MAG3 scintigraphy:

MAG3 is a dynamic marker characterized by its renal uptake and rapid urinary elimination, enabling assessment of the relative function of each kidney and the permeability of the excretory tract (105).

MAG3 scintigraphy should be performed from 4ème or even 5ème weeks of age, due to renal immaturity. It is indicated in the following situations: (108,109)

- Diagnosis of obstructive uropathy: especially in cases of pyelocalic dilatation suggesting pyelocalic junction syndrome. In this case, it may even be performed prior to UCR.
- Follow-up of obstructive uropathies: The aim of this follow-up is to detect any loss of renal function on the same side as the uropathy. In the event of an estimated 10% loss of relative renal function between two examinations, surgical management should be considered.
- Preoperative assessment of obstructive uropathy to better evaluate the degree of obstruction
- Postoperative follow-up of operated uropathy.

1.4. Intravenous urography (IVU):

IVUS is an irradiating examination that allows both a study of the renal parenchyma in search of possible retractive scarring, and a study of the functional capacity of the urinary tract in cases of obstructive uropathy. IVUS is becoming less and less indicated, replaced by scintigraphy, which is less irradiating and more sensitive (22,110).

1.5. Computed tomography (CT):

Renal CT allows us to faithfully reproduce the anatomy of the kidneys and to specify their relationships and vascularization. This information is essential if an excisional procedure is to be considered (111). However, uroscanner has little place in routine paediatric practice, given the technical difficulties involved and the very high radiation exposure (22,112).

1.6. Magnetic resonance imaging (MRI):

MRI enables morphological and functional analysis of the urinary tract in newborns, using fast sequences and sequences taken after injection of Gadolinium.

Rapid sequences are easy to perform in newborns calmed by feeds, without the need for anesthesia. They allow us to study the morphology of the urinary tract, including non-secreting units. The appearance and location of the ureters are sometimes specified.

Longer sequences, repeated over 10 to 20 minutes after gadolinium injection, allow, in conjunction with analysis of enhancement curves as a function of time, assessment of excretory and secretory function. However, in neonates, they are performed under general anaesthetic (113,114).

This is a very promising technique, but it is difficult to access, expensive and requires general anesthesia in newborns, thus limiting its use.

MALFORMATIVE UROPATHIES

1. MALFORMATIVE UROPATHIES (UM) :

1.1. Epidemiology :

Malformative uropathies are congenital anomalies affecting the kidney and excretory tract. Their incidence varies from 5 to 6 ‰ in various studies dating from 1996 onwards, but this estimate underestimates the true frequency of urinary malformations because it does not take into account medical terminations of pregnancy and fetal deaths in utero, which may associate urinary tract malformations in 13 to 20% of cases, and does not include asymptomatic forms of UM discovered at autopsy (115,116).

Several studies carried out in Tunisia have reported a hospital frequency of UM estimated at 4.13 ‰ by Bouchaala (117); at 3.5 ‰ by Kahloul (115) but the exact prevalence of these anomalies remains unknown in Tunisia (115,118).

Urinary tract infection is the most frequent circumstance of discovery, and antenatal ultrasound is becoming increasingly effective in antenatal diagnosis (21).

Internationally, the rate of antenatal screening for UM is in the region of 60-70%, in contrast to developing countries where the rate is no higher than 7%, as the number of ultrasounds performed is still insufficient (115).

A review of the literature shows that the frequency of uropathy in newborns with UTIs ranges from 8% to 26%. (Table XX)

Table IV: Neonatal urinary tract infections and malformative uropathies

Author	Year	UM frequency (%)
Oukkadi (22)	2006	22
Hallab (26)	2006	26
Atmani (3)	2007	26
Sufi (21)	2012	7,5

UM can be divided into two groups: vesico-ureteral reflux, given its frequency and relationship with urinary tract infection, and obstructive uropathy.

1.2. Antenatal diagnosis :

Antenatal diagnosis of malformative uropathies is based on measurement of the anteroposterior diameter of the renal pelvis (renal pelvic diameter). The threshold at which dilatation is considered to have occurred varies from one team to another and according to the term of pregnancy (117,119,120). Several American learned societies have come together to establish a consensus for the definition and classification of dilatation of the urinary tract, based essentially on the Dap of the pelvis on antenatal ultrasound (119,121):

- Low-risk dilatation:
  - ✓ Dap of 4 to 7 mm between 16 and 28 weeks
  - ✓ Dap of 7 to 10 mm after 28 weeks
- Increased-risk dilatation:
  - ✓ Dap ≥7 mm between 16 and 28 weeks
  - ✓ Dap ≥10 mm after 28 weeks

In low-risk fetuses, central calici dilatation may be present, whereas peripheral calici dilatation increases the risk of uropathy. The renal parenchyma should be of normal thickness and appearance, the ureter should not be visible and the bladder should be normal. The presence of unexplained oligohydramnios or peripheral calici dilatation places the fetus in the increased-risk category.

Fetuses are considered at increased risk of postnatal uropathy, based on a DAP of 7 mm at <28 weeks and 10 mm at 28 weeks, or any of the following findings: dilatation of peripheral calyces, renal parenchyma of abnormal thickness or appearance, visibly dilated ureter, abnormal bladder or presence of unexplained oligohydramnios.

Postnatally, to evaluate dilatation detected antenatally, American learned societies recommend 2 ultrasound scans: the first should be performed at least 48 hours after birth, and no later than 1 month. However, in cases of oligohydramnios, urethral obstruction, high-grade bilateral dilatation and concerns about patient compliance with postnatal evaluation, the 1st ultrasound should be performed within the first 48 hours. The second should be performed 1 to 6 months after the first. This period should be shortened to 4-6 weeks in the case of high-risk dilatation.

At the end of this ultrasound, we will have a risk stratification:

- Low risk: Central pyelocalic dilatation with Dap greater than 10 and strictly less than 15 mm
- Moderate risk: Peripheral pyelocalic dilatation with Dap >= 15mm without parenchymal or bladder involvement (ureteral anomalies possible)
- High risk: pyelocalic dilatation and Dap >= 15mm associated with abnormalities of the renal parenchyma and/or bladder

From this risk stratification flow the modalities of management (Table XXI):

Table V: Management strategy according to risk of uropathy

	Low risk	Moderate risk	High risk
Ultrasound follow-up	1-6 months	1-3 months	1 month
UCR	Clinician's decision		Recommended
Antibiotic prophylaxis	Clinician's decision		Recommended
Scintigraphy	Not recommended	Clinician's decision	

According to the European Association of Urology, patients with an antenatal diagnosis of hydronephrosis require 2 ultrasound assessments within the first 2 months of life. The first ultrasound should be performed at D7 of life, due to physiological oliguria. UCR is recommended in cases of high-grade bilateral hydronephrosis, renal duplication with hydronephrosis, ureterocele, ureteral dilatation and urethral anomalies. In all other cases, UCR is optional. When infants with a diagnosis of prenatal hydronephrosis become symptomatic of urinary tract infection, UCR should be considered (122).

1.3. Vesico-ureteral reflux :

Vesico-ureteral reflux is defined as the reflux of urine into the ureter and/or kidney during the filling and/or emptying of the bladder. It remains the most frequent urological anomaly in children.

Its incidence ranges from 0.5% to 3%. The incidence rises to around 30-40% in children with proven and documented UTIs (123,124).

The two main circumstances in which RVU is discovered are urinary tract infection and hydronephrosis on antenatal ultrasound. 15-21% of antenatally diagnosed hydronephrosis is caused by RVU (125,126).

The seriousness of RVU lies in the fact that it predisposes to urinary tract infections, kidney damage leading to hypertension and end-stage renal failure (122).

Therapeutic management is based on 2 approaches: conservative (monitoring and antibiotic prophylaxis) and interventional (endoscopic and surgical treatment).

- Conservative treatment:

Conservative treatment is based on the understanding that VUR can resolve spontaneously as the vesicoureteral junction matures, especially if the reflux is of low intensity. Resolution is close to 80% for grade I-II VUR and 30-50% for grade III-V VUR within 4-5 years of follow-up. Spontaneous resolution is low for high-grade bilateral refluxes (122,127).

The conservative approach includes watchful waiting, intermittent or continuous antibiotic prophylaxis and bladder rehabilitation in patients with lower urinary tract dysfunction (128-130).

Regular clinico-radiological follow-up is part of conservative management to monitor spontaneous resolution and assess renal function. There is no validated monitoring scheme, and the frequency of visits depends on the physician's choice. However, requesting biannual urinary tract ultrasound combined with annual cystography and DMSA scintigraphy (depending on ultrasound and clinical findings) seems reasonable. Conservative management should be questioned in all patients with recurrent urinary tract infections despite prophylaxis, and a more invasive procedure should be considered (122).

With regard to anti-infective prophylaxis, the most frequently used molecules are amoxicillin and trimethoprim for newborns and infants under 2 months of age, and cotrimoxazole and nitrofurantoin for infants over 6 months of age in low single doses (one-third of the curative dose), preferably at bedtime. The use and duration of antibiotic prophylaxis in reflux patients is another area of major controversy (129,131-133).

While some trials show no benefit for continuous antibiotic prophylaxis, particularly in low-grade reflux, other trials show that continuous antibiotic prophylaxis prevents further kidney damage, particularly in patients with grade III and IV reflux (134-137).

The difficulty lies in selecting the group of patients who do not require antibiotic prophylaxis. A number of factors need to be taken into consideration, such as young age, high-grade RVU, toilet-training status, presence of lower urinary tract dysfunction, female gender and male circumcision status, all of which are risk factors for recurrence of urinary tract infection.

A practical approach is to consider antibiotic prophylaxis until children are toilet-trained, and until there is no lower urinary tract dysfunction. Active monitoring of urinary tract infections is necessary after antibiotic prophylaxis has been discontinued (122).

> Endoscopic treatment :

Endoscopic treatment, which is minimally invasive and can be performed on an outpatient basis, is becoming increasingly popular. It involves injecting swelling materials under the ureteral mucosa at the junction between the bladder and the ureter. The swelling agent elevates the ureteral orifice and distal ureter so that coaptation is increased. The narrowed lumen prevents urine reflux, without impeding anterograde urine flow (122). (Figure 26)

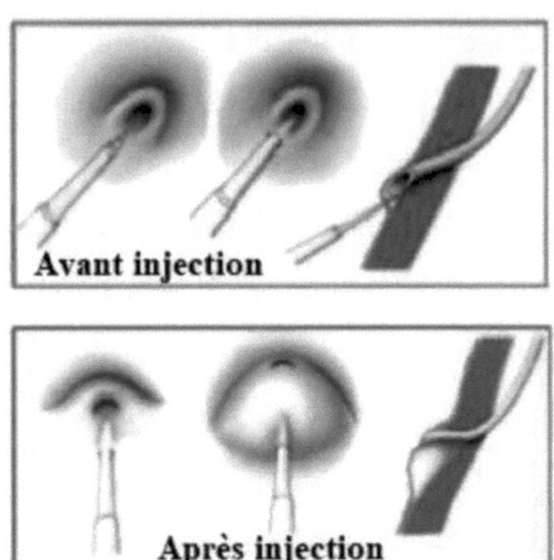

Figure 6: Endoscopic treatment of vesicoureteral reflux

Several substances have been used: polytetrafluoroethylene (PTFE) or Teflon, collagen, autologous fat, polydimethylsiloxane, silicone, chondrocytes and, more recently, a dextranomer/hyaluronic acid solution (Deflux). PTFE was the most effective, but its use in children has not been approved in view of the possible adverse effects of particle migration (138,139). Although other compounds are biocompatible, such as collagen and chondrocytes, these agents have not proved effective.

Deflux was approved in 2001 by the U.S. Food and Drug Administration for the endoscopic treatment of RVU in children.

Early clinical trials demonstrated the efficacy of this agent in the treatment of reflux (140).

In a meta-analysis (141) including 5527 patients and 8101 renal units, the rate of reflux resolution after endoscopic treatment using Deflux was variable according to the grade of Reflux: 78.5% for grades I and II, 72% for grade III, 63% for grade IV, and 51% for grade V.

If the 1st injection failed, the success rate was 68% for the 2nd injection and 34% for the third. The overall success rate with one or more injections was 85%.

Recent prospective randomized trials comparing the efficacy of endoscopic treatment, antibiotic prophylaxis and simple monitoring without antibiotic prophylaxis in 203 infants aged 1 to 2 years with grade III or IV reflux showed that endoscopic treatment had the highest resolution rate, estimated at 71%, compared with 39% for antibiotic prophylaxis and 47% for monitoring at 2-year follow-up. The recurrence rate at 2 years after endoscopic treatment was 20% (142).

The monitoring group had the highest rate of urinary tract infections (57%) and kidney scarring (11%).

- Surgical treatment :

In terms of therapeutic efficacy, surgical cure represents the reference treatment for vesicoureteral reflux in children, with an average success rate of 95% (143,144).

The aim of treatment is to prevent reflux nephropathy or slow its worsening (145).

The main surgical indications for VUR in children are recurrent urinary tract infections, impaired renal function and persistent high-grade vesicoureteral reflux (127,146).

Surgical treatment involves re-implantation of the ureters into the bladder. The aim of treatment is to re-establish a competent valve system by lengthening the submucosal course of the ureter so that it has solid support from the detrusor, enabling occlusion during bladder filling. For the anti-reflux system to function properly, a submucosal pathway corresponding to at least 4 times the ureter's caliber is required. In addition, the ureter must rest on a tonic muscular wall (147).

Several techniques have been reported in the literature, but the one described by Cohen is currently the most widely used (Figure 27). It consists of a trans-trigonal ureteral advancement. The submucosal tunnel extends from the initial meatus to below the contralateral meatus and terminates at the new orifice. In the case of bilateral reflux, the ureters cross over on the midline. In the best hands, the success rate of Cohen's re-implantation technique can be as high as 98%. Post-operative complications are relatively rare, the most serious being stenosis. With Cohen's technique, both ureters can be implanted simultaneously. The disadvantage of this technique is the displacement of the ureteral orifice to the contralateral side, making subsequent endoscopic procedures more difficult (124,125,146).

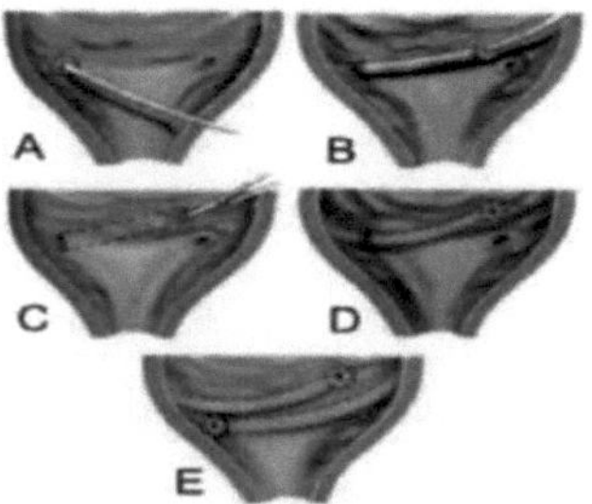

A : incision de la muqueuse périméatique.

B : dissection urétérale par voie endo-vésicale pure

C : tunnélisation sous-muqueuse

D : anastomose urétéro-vésicale

E : anastomose bilatérale croisée

Figure 7: Vesicoureteral reimplantation using Cohen's method

Ureterectomy combined with nephrectomy should be considered in cases of RVU with a destroyed kidney to avoid the risk of infection and hypertension (148).

1.5. Obstructive uropathies:

Obstructive uropathies are due to an obstruction to normal urinary flow that can be caused by a variety of anatomical and functional etiologies.

Common in children, they represent one of the main etiologies of renal failure in children. Treatment relies mainly on surgery to restore good renal drainage. The obstructive uropathies frequently described are (21,149):

- Pyeloureteral junction syndrome: obstruction at the pyeloureteral junction
- Obstructive mega-ureter and ureterocele: obstruction at the vesico-ureteral junction
- Posterior urethral valve: subvesical obstruction

1.4.1. Pyeloureteral junction syndrome:

Pyeloureteral junction syndrome (PJUS) is the most common malformative uropathy in children. It accounts for over 60% of urological anomalies discovered antenatally (21). It is most often unilateral, affecting the left side of the body, and is seen mainly in boys. Children with junction syndrome are generally asymptomatic at birth (150,151).

The etiologies of SJPU are grouped into two groups: primary anomalies in ureteral development (intra-ureteral polyp, narrowing of the lumen due to abnormal collagen development in the wall, atonic ureter) and external compressions (ureteral compression by an inferior polar artery is the classic example being in children) (152).

Ultrasound shows dilated calyces communicating with a dilated pyelon, associated with narrowing at the pyeloureteral junction without ureteral dilatation. In severe cases, renal parenchymal thinning occurs, and in cases of in utero obstruction, renal dysplasia, subcapsular urinoma or urinary ascites may be found. Ultrasound findings in favor of renal dysplasia include parenchymal hyperechogenicity, loss of corticomedullary differentiation and the presence of cortical cysts. Concomitant study of the contralateral kidney is essential to determine whether the obstruction is unilateral or bilateral, to identify any compensatory hypertrophy, and to look for other associated malformations or renal lithiasis (151).

The presence of ureteral dilatation, renal duplicity or bilateral hydronephrosis indicates the need for a UCR to check for associated vesicoureteral reflux or obstruction downstream of the bladder, such as a posterior urethral valve (150). Serum creatinine is also measured (153).

MAG3 scintigraphy allows separate assessment of renal function in each kidney and diagnosis of obstruction (153).

Uro-modensitometry (Uro-CT) may be requested for etiological purposes, in particular to search for a polar vessel crossing the pyeloureteral junction (154).

Biochemical studies of sodium and beta2microglobulin in fetal urine provide precise information on postnatal renal tubular function (155).

Therapeutic management ranges from abstention to surgery. It depends on the stage of hydronephrosis, the degree of tolerance of the obstruction, the age of the child and the degree of sepsis of the urinary tract (156).

Most congenital hydronephrosis regresses spontaneously without intervention. In a prospective randomized trial of infants with unilateral congenital hydronephrosis with DAP> 15 mm and differential function greater than 40%, DAP remained stable in 33% of cases, and spontaneous improvement or resolution was found in 47%.

DAP estimation can guide treatment strategy as follows:

- A DAP of less than 15 mm rarely deteriorates or requires intervention.
- A DAP of between 15 and 30 mm requires regular monitoring.
- A PAD greater than 30 mm has a high probability of surgical management (157).

Surgery is indicated in the following cases:

- Unilateral obstruction associated with a relative renal function of less than 40% of overall renal function or a T1/2 of more than 20 minutes on scintigraphy.
- Worsening of relative renal function exceeding 10% between 2 scan controls.
- Worsening of hydronephrosis on several ultrasound examinations.
- Bilateral pyeloureteral junction syndrome with severe obstruction and parenchymal atrophy (158,159).

The surgical technique of choice is pyeloplasty using the Anderson-Hynes method, which involves excising the stenotic segment and, after spatulation of the ureteral end, creating a wide, watertight anastomosis (157).

1.4.2. Obstructive mega ureter:

The obstructive primary mega ureter is a congenital dilatation of the ureter which lies upstream of a functional obstacle located at the level of the terminal juxtavesical ureter, macroscopically normal with a normal outlet, in a normal bladder, without cervico-urethral obstacle (160,161).

In order of frequency, the mega ureter is the second most common dilatation of the urinary tract discovered antenatally. This uropathy most frequently affects boys, and the left side is its preferred site. Prenatal ultrasonography has improved our understanding of the natural history of uropathies, and revolutionized their management (160).

Brown et al have shown that before the advent of antenatal diagnosis, the mega ureter occupied the 4ème place in terms of frequency of urinary dilatations, after pathology of the pyeloureteral junction (22%), valves of the posterior urethra (19%) and ureterocele (14%), with an estimated frequency of 10% (162).

Post-natal diagnostic confirmation relies mainly on radiological and isotopic examinations of the urinary tract. Renal ultrasound is systematically performed at D5-J7 of life. Its purpose is to confirm the location and extent of ureteral dilatation, measure the diameter of the retrovesical ureter and pyelone and study the state of the renal parenchyma. Ultrasound follow-up is required at around six to eight weeks of age, then every three to six months to monitor progress. Persistent ureteral dilatation greater than 10 mm is a predictive factor for surgery. MAG3 renal scintigraphy, performed from six weeks of age, can be used to assess the impact on renal excretory function, and to determine whether the mega-ureter is obstructive or not. UCR should be performed systematically to detect associated vesico-ureteral reflux, which can worsen the prognosis and justify vesico-ureteral reimplantation (163).

In terms of evolution, primary obstructive mega-ureters regress spontaneously within the first 3 years of life, or remain stable without compromising renal function in 70-80% of cases, justifying a conservative 1st-line approach. Antibiotic prophylaxis may be necessary to protect the kidneys during conservative treatment. Approximately 20% of cases require surgical treatment. In Gimpel's study, 23% of patients benefited from surgical treatment, while only 11.9% of cases in Stehr's study. Indications are recurrent urinary tract infections, renal function impairment of less than 20% and increased ureteral dilatation (163,164).

1.4.3. Posterior urethral valve:

Valves of the posterior urethra are the most common cause of obstructive subvesical syndrome in boys (165). The incidence varies from 1/5000 male births in Perks' study to 1/25000 in Atwel's (166). There are 3 types of VUP according to Young's classification: Type I is the most frequent, found in 95% of cases. (Figure 28)

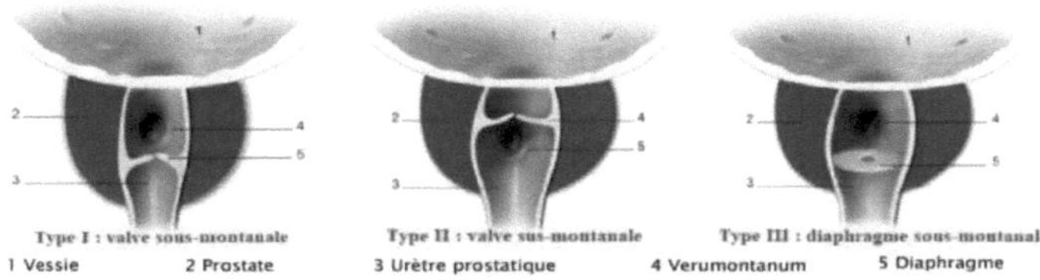

Figure 8: Young's classification

The seriousness of this malformative uropathy lies in its impact on the upper urinary tract, with a significant risk of end-stage renal failure ranging from 25 to 40% (167).

VUPs are diagnosed antenatally in around 18% of cases in Tunisian series. This rate can reach 30% in Western countries.

Ultrasound warning signs are detectable from 20 days' gestation, namely bilateral dilatation of the pyelocalic cavities, a dilated bladder with a thickened, irregular wall, and oligohydramnios (168). Anamnios has a poor prognosis. It reflects an absence of renal filtration, raising fears of secondary pulmonary hypoplasia (166). The sensitivity and specificity of antenatal diagnosis vary according to the degree of obstruction and the presence of associated anomalies (166).

Antenatal diagnosis has made it possible to modify the evolutionary data of this uropathy, with the proposal of medical termination of pregnancy (IMG) in severe cases (168).

In the absence of antenatal diagnosis, the telltale signs vary with age. In the neonatal period, the combination of an abnormally hard bladder, dripping micturition and a poor urine stream is the most constant sign. The diagnosis should also be made in the presence of urinary tract infection, urinary ascites or dehydration with anorexia and vomiting (165).

Radiological investigations are essentially based on ultrasound and UCR, which reveal direct and indirect signs of the valves. UCR can also show an associated RVU in 65% of cases, bilateral in 50%. In 25% to 50% of cases, these UCRs disappear following removal of the urethral obstruction (169,170).

Radical treatment of VUP is based on resection of the valve, which can be performed endoscopically. Pending resection, emergency bladder drainage is indicated in cases of retention, usually via a urethral catheter, less frequently via a suprapubic catheter. Upper tract drainage by percutaneous nephrostomy is indicated in cases of sepsis and/or renal failure, to relieve the kidneys of hyperpressure and subsequently improve renal function (170).

TREATMENT

1. TREATMENT :

1.1. Curative treatment :

The high risk of bacterial dissemination in newborns, the lack of knowledge of the anatomical state of the urinary tract during a first infectious episode, and the frequency of association with malformative uropathies, particularly RVU, make neonatal urinary tract infection a genuine therapeutic emergency.

The aim of treatment is to sterilize urine and renal parenchyma, avoid bacterial dissemination, prevent recurrence and prevent the occurrence of renal scarring and long-term chronic renal failure (26,171).

Antibiotics used in the treatment of urinary tract infections (UTIs) must meet a number of criteria: rapid bactericidal action, very high urinary and renal concentration (8 to 10 times the MIC) to eradicate intra-parenchymal deposits, and renal elimination in active form at high concentration (98).

Empirical antibiotic therapy must take into account the resistance profile of the most common urinary tract germs (172).

3rd-generation cephalosporins are most often active on the majority of germs encountered in urinary tract infections, notably E.coli and other enterobacteria (173).

Cefotaxime is the drug of choice. Ceftriaxone is contraindicated in premature infants with a post-menstrual age of less than 41 weeks, in full-term neonates with hyperbilirubinemia, due to the risk of altered bilirubin binding, and in infusion of calcium-containing solutions, due to the risk of precipitation of a calcium salt of ceftriaxone (174).

Cefotaxime-aminoside dual therapy provides a synergistic effect, increasing the rate of bactericidal action and reducing the emergence of resistant strains (175).

Enterobacteriaceae resistant to extended-spectrum β-lactamase (ESBL) production have been on the rise in recent years (98,176). Carbapenems are the reference treatment for infections with ESBL bacteria, found mainly in hospitals (176,177), but they also encourage the emergence of even more resistant strains, through the production of carbapenemases (106). Aminoglycosides remain active in most cases of this type of infection (176).

Hospitalization is systematic for newborns (79,99,178).

Antibiotic therapy is administered parenterally, combining cefotaxime 100 mg/kg/day and an aminoglycoside gentamicin 5 mg/kg/day or amikacin 15 mg/kg/day. The recommended duration of dual therapy is 4-5 days, with cefotaxime administered for 10 days.

Recognition of associated meningitis implies doubling the dose of betalactamine and extending the duration of treatment to 21 days (175).

A retrospective Spanish study by Magin et al. of neonates with urinary tract infections. Cases of associated meningitis were excluded. These neonates were treated with dual therapy (betalactamine + gentamicin) for an average of 4 days parenterally, with oral relay, and showed no evidence of therapeutic failure or recurrence (179). For this reason, the new Swiss recommendations for the treatment of urinary tract infections in newborns indicate an initial parenteral treatment with oral relay depending on the results of the urine culture antibiogram, preferably with a targeted monotherapy. In the event of sepsis with bacteremia, consideration should be given to extending the duration of parenteral treatment. In the event of inadequate response to intravenous treatment, vomiting or eating disorders, oral therapy should not be continued. In children with acute and/or chronic renal disease, severe renal or urological malformation or neurological bladder, intravenous treatment should be considered, and the decision to switch to the oral route should be discussed with the nephrologist, urologist and paediatric infectious diseases specialist (99).

1.2. Preventive treatment :

Preventive treatment is essentially based on hygiene measures and antibiotic prophylaxis.

1.2.1. Hygiene measures :

Hygiene measures for newborns are extrapolated from those recommended for infants and older children.

- Good hydration is recommended to ensure frequent and complete micturition, as the regular emptying of the bladder ensures the sterility of the urine.
- Perineal cleansing with soap and water once a day, as too little or too much cleansing can disrupt the bacterial flora and encourage the development of intestinal germs.
- Wipe from front to back
- Phimosis predisposes to urinary tract infections. In the event of recurrent urinary tract infections with phimosis, it is advisable to apply a steroid cream twice a day (180,181).

1.2.2. Antibiotic prophylaxis:

Antibiotics used to prevent urinary tract infections must meet certain criteria:

- be active against the most common uropathogenic germs
- be orally active
- be excreted in sufficient concentration in the urine in native form,
- be well tolerated and not conducive to the emergence of resistant strains
- ensure compliance

Preventive doses are much lower than curative doses, in the order of 20-30% of those recommended for curative treatment. A single daily dose, preferably in the evening, is usually sufficient, as it allows the antibiotics to stagnate overnight in the bladder (21,180).

Betalactam antibiotics and quinolones are not recommended, as they encourage the emergence of resistant mutants. An exception is made for neonates, in whom the use of amoxicillin is authorized (99).

Several drugs belonging to different classes of antibiotics have been evaluated in children in terms of long-term efficacy and safety: (39,99,181,182)

- Cotrimoxazole (Bactrim®): This is the most widely used and studied antibiotic for long-term urinary prophylaxis in children. The dose recommended by the Société Française de Néphrologie Pédiatrique is 10 mg/kg/d for sulfamethoxazole and 2 mg/kg/d for trimethoprim, taken once daily.

It is contraindicated in premature babies and newborns under 1 month of age.

Cotrimoxazole has no impact on intestinal flora. It is well tolerated and rarely causes side effects.

- Nitrofurantoin (Furadoïne®, Furadantine®): no longer authorized for pediatric use in France since 1999, following the discovery of a mutagenic tendency in animals. However, some teams continue to prescribe it at a dose of 1 to 2 mg/kg/day, as a single dose.

Nitrofurantoin does not lead to the emergence of resistant strains in the faecal flora. Its adverse effects, namely nausea and vomiting, lead to discontinuation of treatment in certain cases. Nitrofurantoin is contraindicated in newborns under 1 month of age.

- Nitroxoline (Nibiol®) is prescribed at a dose of 10 mg/kg/day. The oral suspension is no longer marketed, limiting its use in small children. This molecule has marketing authorization for children over 6 years of age.

- Amoxicillin (Clamoxyl® and generics) can be used for infants under 2 months of age at a dose of 20mg/kg/D in twice-daily doses. In view of the emergence of resistant strains, its use in this indication should be discussed (40% of E. coli strains isolated in towns and cities in France are resistant to amoxicillin).

- Cefaclor (Alfatil® and generics): belongs to the 1st-generation cephalosporin family. It is indicated in particular for newborns and infants with antenatal diagnosis of malformative uropathy, at a dose of 3 to 5 mg/kg/day taken daily, and is well tolerated. It is a more recent molecule, but prospective studies in this indication are almost non-existent.

- Cefixime (Oroken® and generics): belongs to the 3rd-generation cephalosporin family. The recommended dose is 2mg/kg/d in 1 daily dose. It is contraindicated in premature babies and newborns.

Antibiotic prophylaxis remains a controversial topic in the literature, with many confusing data. Has it proven effective? Should antibiotic prophylaxis be continuous, sequential or intermittent? What is the ideal duration and when should antibiotic prophylaxis be discontinued?

1.2.3. Surgical prevention: circumcision :

The foreskin is colonized during infancy and early childhood by bacteria including strains of *Proteus mirabilis, Pseudomonas* species, *Klebsiella, Serratia* and *Escherichia coli*, which can cause urinary tract infections in newborns (183).

According to a meta-analysis by Singh-Grewal et al, including a randomized trial and 11 observational studies, the prevalence of urinary tract infections is reduced by 90% in circumcised infants. In a more recent meta-analysis of 14 studies by Skaikh et al, the prevalence of febrile UTIs in infants under three months of age was 7.5% in girls, 2.4% in circumcised boys and 20.1% in uncircumcised boys.

It is estimated that preventing a single urinary tract infection requires the circumcision of 111 to 125 normal newborns. In higher-risk boys with recurrent UTIs or underlying uropathy, circumcision may be more beneficial (184).

EVOLUTION

1. EVOLUTION :

1.1. Immediate development :

The clinical course may be favorable, with apyrexia achieved by the 2nd-3rd day and disappearance of the biological inflammatory syndrome by the end of treatment (21). A follow-up ECBU is no longer recommended in this case (185,186).

If there is no clinical improvement after 48-72 hours, the patient should be investigated for complications such as renal abscesses, primary or secondary antibiotic resistance, or other localization of the infection (79,187).

1.2. Recurrences :

The rate of recurrence of urinary tract infection, within 6 to 12 months of the first episode, varies between 20% and 48% in different studies (188). In Anoukoum's series, 16% of children had experienced a recurrence (189).

1.3. Long-term trend :

Aggression of the renal parenchyma can lead to renal scarring, which in turn can lead to hypertension or renal failure. This risk is related to the delay in treatment and the presence of malformative uropathy. The higher the risk, the earlier the first episode of UTI, particularly in the neonatal period (190-192). The incidence of renal scarring after UTI varies from region to region, ranging from 26.5% in Australia to 49% in Asia (193). The presence of associated vesico-ureteral reflux increases the risk of post-infectious renal scarring (193). These scars are associated with an estimated 10% risk of developing chronic renal failure in adulthood (21). According to Manich et al, in the presence of post-infectious renal lesions, the risk of developing hypertension can be as high as 26%. This risk is increased in the presence of bilateral or extensive renal scarring, bilateral RVU and in males. Long-term follow-up is therefore essential (190). In the absence of a consensus, annual blood pressure measurement and annual screening for microalbuminuria may be sufficient (194).

CONCLUSION

Urinary tract infection is a frequent pathology in newborns. Knowing how to diagnose it early and treat it appropriately helps prevent kidney scarring and the progression to hypertension and renal failure.

Early and appropriate treatment of neonatal UTI could prevent the development of parenchymal lesions and reduce long-term morbidity. We therefore propose a management protocol for urinary tract infection in neonates:

1- Preventive care :

Preventive management is based on hygienic-dietary rules and the management of malformative uropathies discovered during antenatal ultrasound.

- Hygienic and dietary measures :
  - Good hydration is recommended to ensure frequent and complete micturition, as the regular emptying of the bladder ensures the sterility of the urine.
  - Perineal cleansing with soap and water once a day, as too little or too much cleansing can disrupt the bacterial flora and encourage the development of intestinal germs.
  - Wipe from front to back
  - Phimosis predisposes to urinary tract infections. In the event of a recurrence of urinary tract infection with phimosis, it is advisable to apply a steroid cream twice a day.
- Management of urinary tract dilatations discovered on antenatal ultrasound :

In the event of antenatal discovery of urinary tract dilatation, renal ultrasound should be performed at D5-J7 of life, or within the first 48 hours of life in cases of severe urinary tract dilatation, suspected posterior urethral valve, bilateral dilatation or single kidney dilatation.

At the end of this ultrasound examination, management will be guided according to the pyelic DAP and associated urinary tract abnormalities on ultrasound.

(Figure 29)

- Management of the main uropathies diagnosed in the neonatal period :

We have attempted to establish a management protocol for the most common uropathies: vesicoureteral reflux (Figure 30), posterior urethral valve (Figure 31), junction syndrome (Figure 32) and obstructive mega ureter (Figure 33).

2- Curative management :

- Systematic hospitalization
- Bacteriological confirmation: ECBU
- Biological work-up: CBC, CRP and creatinine.
- Blood culture followed by intravenous dual therapy with cefotaxime + aminoglycoside for 5 days
- Relay per os according to antibiogram results, except in cases of insufficient response to intravenous treatment (vomiting or eating disorders) and in children with acute and/or chronic renal disease, severe renal or urological malformations.
- Total duration of treatment: 10 days (excluding complications or associated meningitis)
- Systematic renal ultrasonography: at a distance from the UTI or

after 48 hours of treatment: in the event of sepsis, oliguria, deterioration in renal function or absence of clinical improvement after 48 hours of treatment.

- UCR as soon as possible in case of atypical urinary tract infection, recurrent urinary tract infection, abnormalities on renal ultrasound or family history of vesico-ureteral reflux.
- DMSA scintigraphy: after the infectious episode of 4 to 6 months: in case of atypical or recurrent urinary tract infection, or in case of ultrasound abnormalities
- MAG3 scintigraphy for suspected obstructive uropathy

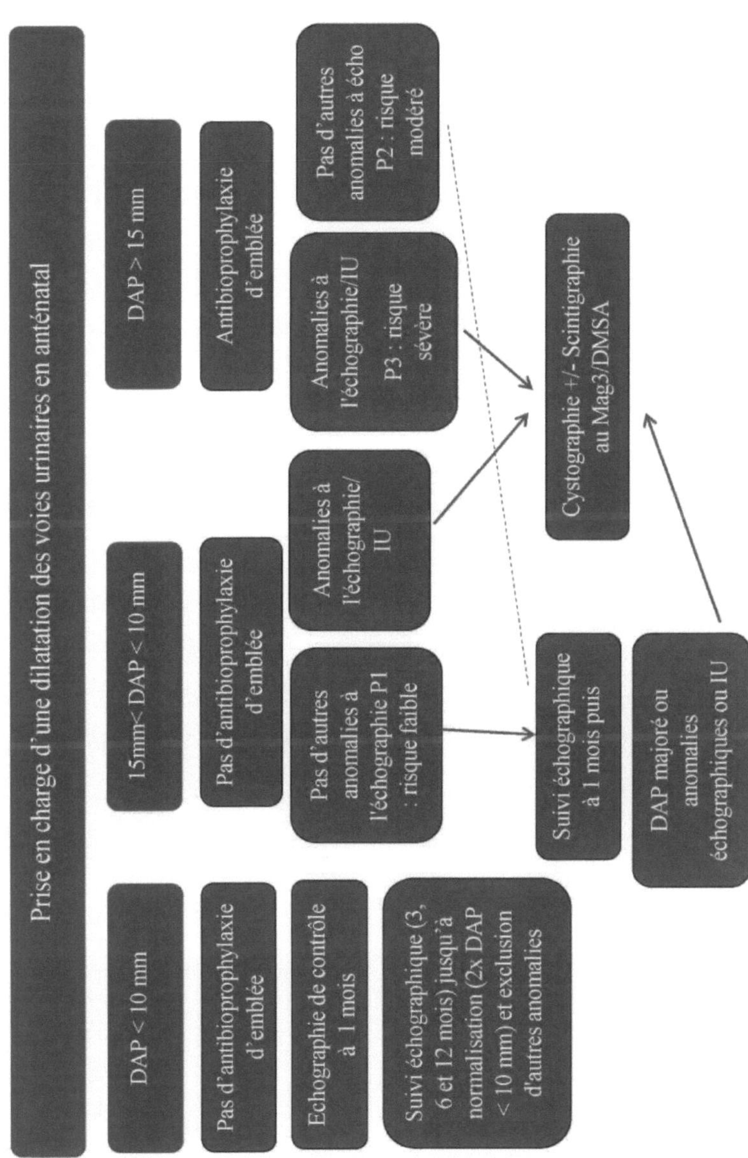

Figure 9: Management protocol for antenatal urinary tract dilatation

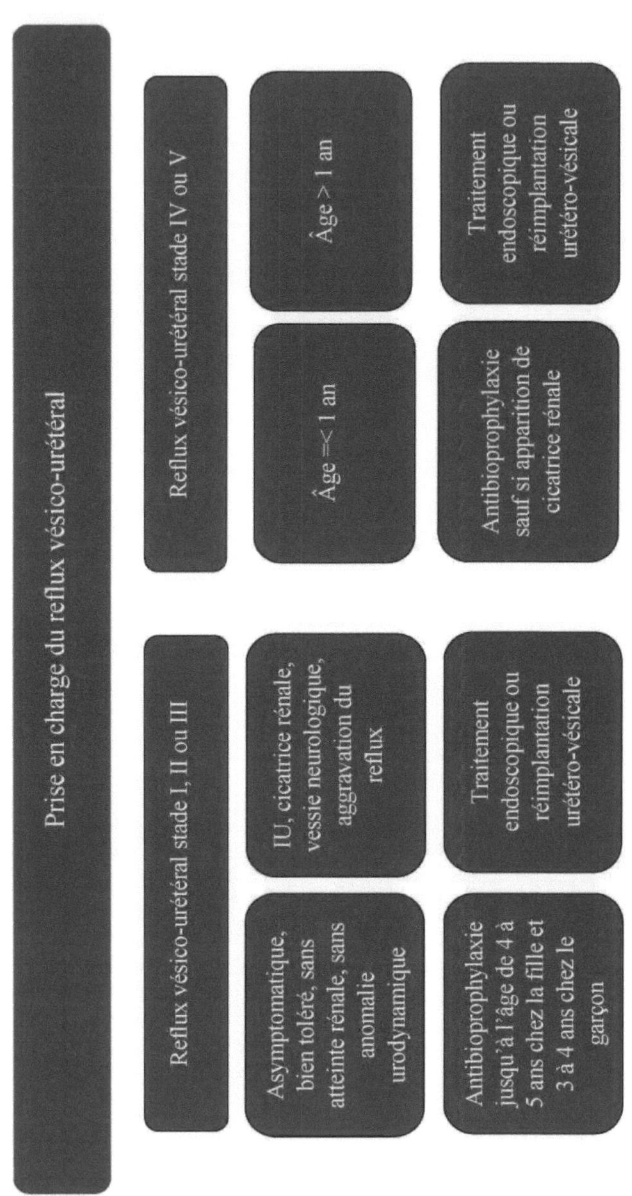

Figure 10: Vesicoureteral reflux management protocol

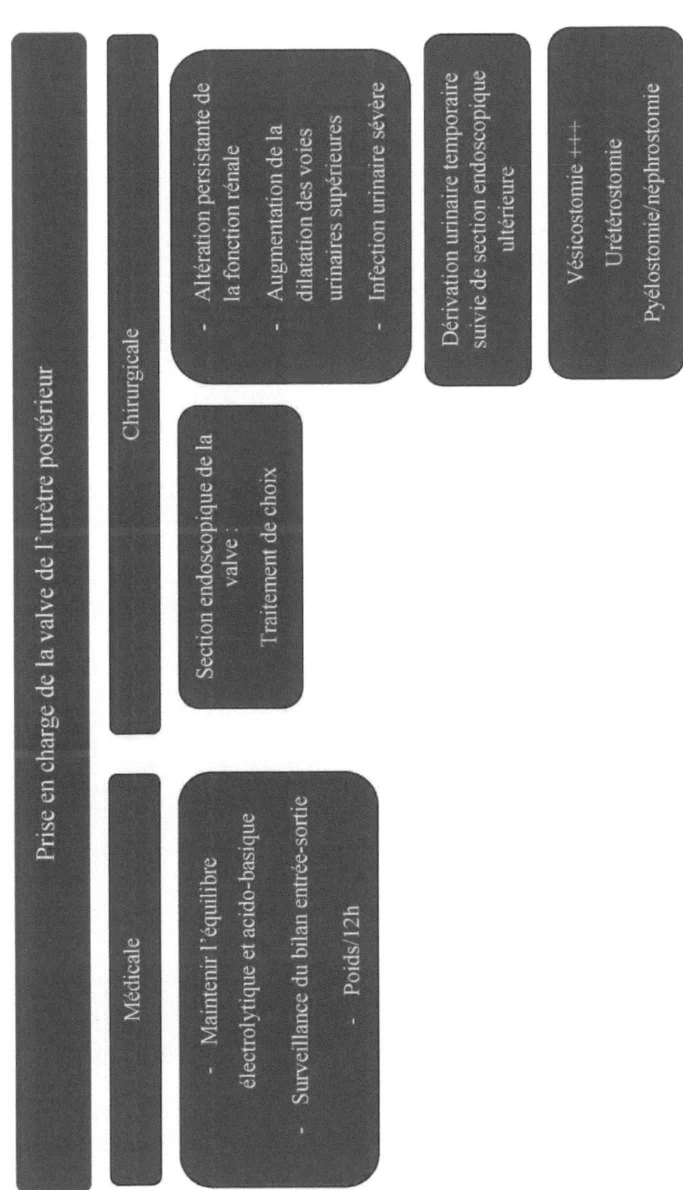

Figure 11: Posterior urethral valve management protocol

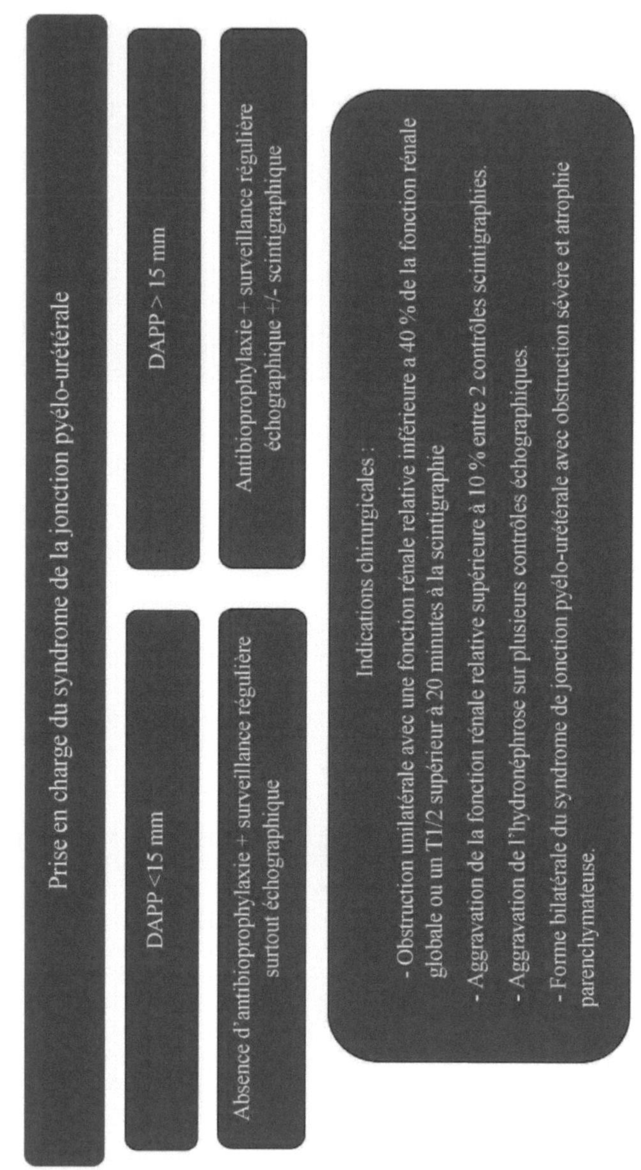

Figure 12: Management protocol for pyeloureteral junction syndrome

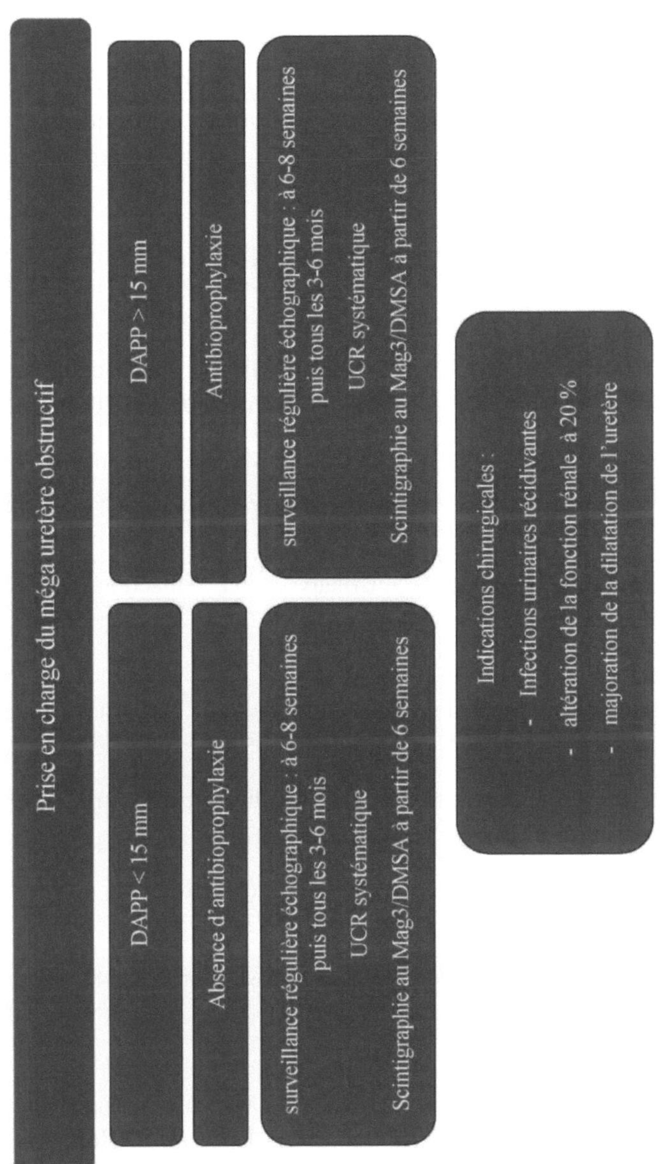

Figure 13: Management protocol for obstructive mega ureters

REFERENCES

1. López Sastre JB, Ramos Aparicio A, Coto Cotallo GD, Fernández Colomer B, Crespo Hernández M. Urinary tract infection in the newborn: clinical and radio imaging studies. Pediatric Nephrology. 2007;22(10):1735-41.

2. Youssef D, Elfateh H, Sedeek R, Seleem S. Epidemiology of urinary tract infection in neonatal intensive care unit: A single center study in Egypt. Journal of Academy of Medical Sciences. 2012;2(1):25.

3. Atmani S, Aouragh R, Bouharrou A, Hida M. Neonatal urinary tract infection: about 23 cases. J Pediatr Pueric. 2007 Apr;20(2):70-3.

4. Gérard M, Diakite B, Bedu A, Titti I, Mariani-Kurkdjian P, Lotmann H, et al. L'infection urinaire du nouveau-né. Archives de Pédiatrie. 1998 Jan;5:254S-259S.

5. BEGUE.P; S.BARON. Urinary tract infection. Pathologies infectieuses de l'enfant. 1988. p. 340-1.

6. Sarici SU, Kul M, Alpay F. Neonatal Jaundice Coinciding With or Resulting From Urinary Tract Infections? Pediatrics. 2003 Nov 1;112(5):1212-3.

7. Dumas R. Urinary tract infections: paediatric particularities. Rev Prat. 1990;40(29):2763-6.

8. Bergstrom T, Larson H, Winberg J. Studies of urinary tract infections in infancy and childhood. J Pediatr. 1972 May;80(5):855-7.

9. Tripathi S, Malik G. Neonatal Sepsis: past, present and future; a review article. Internet Journal of Medical Update - EJOURNAL. 2010 Jul 6;5(2):45-54.

10. Riskin A, Toropine A, Bader D, Hemo M, Srugo I, Kugelman A. Is it Justified to Include Urine Cultures in Early (< 72 Hours) Neonatal Sepsis Evaluations of Term and Late Preterm Infants? Am J Perinatol. 2012 Nov 12;30(06):499-504.

11. Kaufman J, Temple-Smith M, Sanci L. Urinary tract infections in

children: an overview of diagnosis and management. BMJ Paediatr Open. 2019 Sep 24;3(1).

12. Lin CW, Chiou YH, Chen YY, Huang YF, Hsieh KS, Sung PK. Urinary Tract Infection in Neonates. Clinical Neuroscience. 1999;6(2):1-4.

13. Shaw KN, Gorelick M, McGowan KL, Yakscoe NM, Schwartz JS. Prevalence of Urinary Tract Infection in Febrile Young Children in the Emergency Department. Pediatrics. 1998 August 1;102(2):e16-e16.

14. Cataldi L, Zaffanello M, Gnarra M, Fanos V. Urinary tract infection in the newborn and the infant: state of the art. The Journal of Maternal-Fetal & Neonatal Medicine. 2010 Oct;23(S3):90-3.

15. Bonadio W, Maida G. Urinary Tract Infection in Outpatient Febrile Infants Younger than 30 Days of Age. Pediatric Infectious Disease Journal. 2014 Apr;33(4):342-4.

16. Ismaili K, Lolin K, Damry N, Alexander M, Lepage P, Hall M. Febrile Urinary Tract Infections in 0- to 3-Month-Old Infants: A Prospective Follow-Up Study. J Pediatr. 2011 Jan;158(1):91-4.

17. Downey LC, Benjamin DK, Clark RH, Watt KM, Hornik CP, Laughon MM, et al. Urinary tract infection concordance with positive blood and cerebrospinal fluid cultures in the neonatal intensive care unit. Journal of Perinatology. 2013 Apr 30;33(4):302-6.

18. Littlewood JM. 66 Infants with Urinary Tract Infection in First Month of Life. Arch Dis Child. 1972 Apr 1;47(252):218-26.

19. Capdevila Cogul E, Martín Ibáñez I, Mainou Cid C, Toral Rodríguez E, Cols Roig Mf, Agut Quijano T, et al. First urinary tract infection in healthy infants: epidemiology, diagnosis and treatment. An Esp Pediatr. 2001 Oct;55(4):310-4.

20. Iacobelli S, Bonsante F, Guignard JP. Urinary tract infections in pediatrics. Archives de Pédiatrie. 2009 Jul;16(7):1073-9.

21. Soufi M. Urinary tract infection in newborns. Thesis for doctorate in medicine. Sousse Faculty of Medicine; 2012.

22. Oukkadi A. Urinary tract infection of the newborn: A propos de 54 cases. Thèse de doctorat en médecine. Faculty of Medicine, Monastir; 2006.

23. Leumann EP. Urinary tract infections in infants and children. Med Hyg (Geneve). 1989;47:3101-6.

24. Piot M, Chouraqui JP, François JP, et al. Diagnosis of urinary tract infection in the neonatal period. Méd Infant. 1982;89(5):519-28.

25. Sayah A. Urinary tract infections in the neonatal period. Thesis for doctorate in medicine. Faculty of Medicine, Sousse; 1997.

26. Hallab L. Newborn urinary tract infections (89 cases). Doctoral thesis in medicine. Faculté De Médecine Et De Pharmacie de Casablanca; 2006.

27. Dechelette E, François P, Baudain P, Joannard A, Prost-Celse MH, Bost M. L'infection urinaire du nouveau-né à propos de 140 cas. Clinical, bacteriological and radiological study. J Agrégés. 1980;12:485-92.

28. Bilgen H, Ozek E, Unver T, Biyikli N, Alpay H, Cebeci D. Urinary tract infection and hyperbilirubinemia. Turk J Pediatr. 2006;48(1):51-5.

29. Xinias I, Demertzidou V, Mavroudi A, Kollios K, Kardaras P, Papachristou F, et al. Bilirubin levels predict renal cortical changes in jaundiced neonates with urinary tract infection. World Journal of Pediatrics. 2009 Feb 21;5(1):42-5.

30. Mutlu M, Çayir Y, Asian Y. Urinary tract infections in neonates with jaundice in their first two weeks of life. World Journal of Pediatrics. 2014 May 21;10(2):164-7.

31. Ozcan M, Sarici SÜ, Yurdugül Y, Akpinar M, Altun D, Ozcan B, et al. Association Between Early Idiopathic Neonatal Jaundice and Urinary Tract Infections. Clin Med Insights Pediatr. 2017;11.

32. Naveh Y, Friedman A. Urinary tract infection presenting with jaundice. Pediatrics. 1978 Oct;62(4):524-5.

33. Perrin LP. Icterus after urinary tract infection in neonates. Thesis for doctorate in medicine. Faculty of Medicine, Limoges; 1994.

34. Biyikli NK, Alpay H, Ozek E, Akman I, Bilgen H. Neonatal urinary tract infections: Analysis of the patients and recurrences. Pediatrics International. 2004 Feb;46(1):21-5.

35. Bauer S, Eliakim A, Pomeranz A, Regev R, Litmanovits I, Arnon S, et al. Urinary tract infection in very low birth weight preterm infants. Pediatric Infectious Disease Journal. 2003 May;22(5):426-9.

36. Mathieu H. Urinary tract infection. Néphrologie pédiatrique, Flammarion, médecine science, Paris1983 :133-55.

37. Janvier F, Mbongo-Kama E, Mérens A, Cavallo JD. Les difficultés d'interprétation de l'examen cytobactériologique des urines. Revue Francophone des Laboratoires. 2008 nov;2008(406):51-9.

38. Courcol R, Marmonier A, Piemont Y. Les difficultés d'interprétat ion de l'examen cyto-bactériologique des urines. Revue Française des Laboratoires. 2005 Feb;2005(370):21-5.

39. American Academy of Pediatrics Committee on Quality Improvement. Subcommittee on Urinary Tract Infection. Practice parameter: the diagnosis, treatment, and evaluation of the initial urinary tract infection in febrile infants and young children. Pediatrics. 1999;103(4):843-52.

40. Lamy C, Blanc P. Urine sampling: from recommendations to practice, what impact on children's pain? In: 19e Journées La douleur de l'enfant Quelles réponses? 2012. p. 111-7.

41. Rao S. A new urine collection method; pad and moisture sensitive alarm. Arch Dis Child. 2003 Sep 1;88(9):836-836.

42. Diviney J, Jaswon MS. Urine collection methods and dipstick testing in nontoilet-trained children. Pediatric Nephrology. 2021 Jul 12;36(7):1697-708.

43. Hadjipanayis A, Grossman Z, del Torso S, van Esso D, Dornbusch HJ, Mazur A, et al. Current primary care management of children aged 1-36 months with urinary tract infections in Europe: large scale survey

of paediatric practice. Arch Dis Child. 2015 Apr;100(4):341-7.

44. Newman TB, Bernzweig JA, Takayama JI, Finch SA, Wasserman RC, Pantell RH. Urine Testing and Urinary Tract Infections in Febrile Infants Seen in Office Settings. Arch Pediatr Adolesc Med. 2002 Jan 1;156(1):44-54.

45. Alam MT, Coulter JBS, Pacheco J, Correia JB, Ribeiro MGB, Coelho MFC, et al. Comparison of urine contamination rates using three different methods of collection: clean-catch, cotton wool pad and urine bag. Ann Trop Paediatr. 2005 March 18;25(1):29-34.

46. Liaw LCT. Home collection of urine for culture from infants by three methods: survey of parents' preferences and bacterial contamination rates. BMJ. 2000 May 13;320(7245):1312-3.

47. Feasey S. Are Newcastle urine collection pads suitable as a means of collecting specimens from infants? Paediatr Nurs. 1999 nov 1;11(9): 17-21.

48. Macfarlane PI, Ellis R, Hughes C, Houghton C, Lord R. Urine collection pads: are samples reliable for urine biochemistry and microscopy? Pediatric Nephrology. 2005 Feb 28;20(2):170-9.

49. Vernon S, Redfearn A, Pedler SJ, Lambert HJ, Coulthard MG. Urine collection on sanitary towels. The Lancet. 1994 Aug;344(8922):612.

50. Ahmad T, Vickers D, Campbell S, Coulthard MG, Pedler S. Urine collection from disposable nappies. The Lancet. 1991 Sep;338(8768):674-6.

51. Rao S. A new urine collection method; pad and moisture sensitive alarm. Arch Dis Child. 2003 Sep 1;88(9):836-836.

52. Butler CC, Sterne JAC, Lawton M, O'Brien K, Wootton M, Hood K, et al. Nappy pad urine samples for investigation and treatment of UTI in young children: The "DUTY" prospective diagnostic cohort study. British Journal of General Practice. 2016 Jul 1;66(648):e516-24.

53. Hay AD, Birnie K, Busby J, Delaney B, Downing H, Dudley J, et al. The Diagnosis of Urinary Tract infection in Young children (DUTY):

a prospective diagnostic observational study to derive and validate a clinical algorithm for the diagnosis of urinary tract infection in children presenting to primary care with an acute illness. Health Technol Assess (Rockv). 2016 Jul;20(51):1-294.

54. Altuntas N, Celebi Tayfur A, Kocak M, Razi HC, Akkurt S. Midstream clean-catch urine collection in newborns: a randomized controlled study. Eur J Pediatr. 2015 May 1;174(5):577-82.

55. Macfarlane PI, Houghton C, Hughes C. Pad urine collection for ear ly childhood urinary-tract infection. The Lancet. 1999 Aug;354(9178):571.

56. Tosif S, Baker A, Oakley E, Donath S, Babl FE. Contamination rates of different urine collection methods for the diagnosis of urinary tract infections in young children: An observational cohort study. J Paediatr Child Health. 2012 Aug;48(8):659-64.

57. Ho IVA, Lee CH, Fry M. A prospective comparative pilot study comparing the urine collection pad with clean catch urine technique in non-toilet- trained children. Int Emerg Nurs. 2014 Apr;22(2):94-7.

58. Teo S, Cheek JA, Craig S. Improving clean-catch contamination rates: A prospective interventional cohort study. EMA - Emergency Medicine Australasia. 2016 Dec 1;28(6):698-703.

59. Tosif S, Kaufman J, Fitzpatrick P, Hopper SM, Hoq M, Donath S, et al. Clean catch urine collection: Time taken and diagnostic implication. A prospective observational study. J Paediatr Child Health. 2017 Oct;53(10):970-5.

60. Herreros Fernandez ML, Gonzalez Merino N, Tagarro Garcia A, Perez Seoane B, de la Serna Martinez M, Contreras Abad MT, et al. A new technique for fast and safe collection of urine in newborns. Arch Dis Child. 2013 Jan 1;98(1):27-9.

61. Kumar R, . N, Rudrappa S. Mid-stream clean catch urine collection in newborns: a non-invasive and safe technique. Int J Contemp Pediatrics. 2019 Feb 23;6(2):349.

62. Labrosse M, Levy A, Autmizguine J, Gravel J. Evaluation of a new strategy for clean-catch urine in infants. Pediatrics. 2016 Sep 1;138(3).

63. Valleix-Leclerc M, Bahans C, Tahir A, Faubert S, Fargeot A, Abouchi S, et al. Prospective evaluation of a bladder stimulation technique to induce micturition in non-continental children. Archives de Pediatrie. 2016 August 1;23(8):815-9.

64. Kaufman J, Fitzpatrick P, Tosif S, Hopper SM, Donath SM, Bryant PA, et al. Faster clean catch urine collection (Quick-Wee method) from infants: Randomised controlled trial. BMJ. 2017;357.

65. Weill O, Labrosse M, Levy A, Desjardins MP, Trottier ED, Gravel J. Point-of-care ultrasound before attempting clean-catch urine collection in infants: A randomized controlled trial. Canadian Journal of Emergency Medicine. 2019 Sep 1;21(5):646-52.

66. Raymond J, Sauvestre C. Microbiological diagnosis of urinary tract infections in children. Interest of rapid tests. Archives de Pédiatrie. 1998 Jan;5:260S-265S.

67. Eliacik K, Kanik A, Yavascan O, Alparslan C, Kocyigit C, Aksu N, et al. A Comparison of Bladder Catheterization and Suprapubic Aspiration Methods for Urine Sample Collection From Infants With a Suspected Urinary Tract Infection. Clin Pediatr (Phila). 2016 Aug;55(9):819-24.

68. Kozer E, Rosenbloom E, Goldman D, Lavy G, Rosenfeld N, Goldman M. Pain in Infants Who Are Younger Than 2 Months During Suprapubic Aspiration and Transurethral Bladder Catheterization: A Randomized, Controlled Study. Pediatrics. 2006 Jul 1;118(1):e51-6.

69. Watson AR. Urinary tract infection in early childhood. Journal of Antimicrobial Chemotherapy. 1994 August 1;34(suppl A):53-60.

70. McTaggart S, Danchin M, Ditchfield M, Hewitt I, Kausman J, Kennedy S, et al. KHA-CARI guideline: Diagnosis and treatment of urinary tract infection in children. Nephrology. 2015 Feb;20(2):55-60.

71. Ammenti A, Alberici I, Brugnara M, Chimenz R, Guarino S, la Manna

A, et al. Updated Italian recommendations for the diagnosis, treatment and follow-up of the first febrile urinary tract infection in young children. Vol. 109, Acta Paediatrica, International Journal of Paediatrics. Blackwell Publishing Ltd; 2020. p. 236-47.

72. Roberts KB, Downs SM, Finnell SME, Hellerstein S, Shortliffe LD, Wald ER, et al. Urinary tract infection: Clinical practice guideline for the diagnosis and management of the initial UTI in febrile infants and children 2 to 24 months. Vol. 128, Pediatrics. 2011. p. 595-610.

73. Peniakov M, Antonelli J, Naor O, Miron D. Reduction in Contamination of Urine Samples Obtained by In-Out Catheterization by Culturing the Later Urine Stream. Pediatr Emerg Care. 2004 June;20(6):418-9.

74. Karacan C, Erkek N, Senel S, Akin Gunduz S, Catli G, Tavil B. Evaluation of urine collection methods for the diagnosis of urinary tract infection in children. Medical Principles and Practice. 2010 March;19(3):188-91.

75. Al-Orifi F, McGillivray D, Tange S, Kramer MS. Urine culture from bag specimens in young children: Are the risks too high? J Pediatr. 2000 Aug;137(2):221-6.

76. Herreros ML, Tagarro A, García-Pose A, Sánchez A, Cañete A, Gili P. Accuracy of a new clean-catch technique for diagnosis of urinary tract infection in infants younger than 90 days of age. Paediatr Child Health. 2015 August 1;20(6):e30-2.

77. Mori R, Lakhanpaul M, Verrier-Jones K. Diagnosis and management of urinary tract infection in children: summary of NICE guidance. BMJ. 2007 Aug 25;335(7616):395-7.

78. Pezzlo M. Laboratory diagnosis of urinary tract infections: Guidelines, challenges, and innovations. Clin Microbiol Newsl. 2014 June 15;36(12):87-93.

79. Urinary tract infection in under 16s: diagnosis and management NICE guideline. 2022.

80. Dosquet P. Leukocyturia-bacteriuria: diagnostic orientation. Rev Part. 1992;42(9):1193-4.

81. Kurul §, Simons SHP, Ramakers CRB, de Rijke YB, Kornelisse RF, Reiss IKM, et al. Association of inflammatory biomarkers with subsequent clinical course in suspected late onset sepsis in preterm neonates. Crit Care. 2021 Dec 6;25(1):12.

82. Reinhart K, Meisner M, Brunkhorst FM. Markers for Sepsis Diagnosis: What is Useful? Crit Care Clin. 2006 Jul;22(3):503-19.

83. Weitkamp JH, Aschner JL. Diagnostic Use of C-Reactive Protein (CRP) in Assessment of Neonatal Sepsis. Neoreviews. 2005 Nov 1;6(11):e508-15.

84. Gendrel D. Urinary tract infection and biological markers: C-reactive protein, interleukins and procalcitonin. Archives de Pédiatrie. 1998 Jan;5:269S- 273S.

85. Heches X, Pignol M, van Ditzhuyzen O, Koffi B. Interleukin 6 or interleukin 8? An aid to early diagnosis of bacterial infection in newborns less than 12 hours old. Immunoanalysis & Specialized Biology. 2000 Sept;15(5):346-53.

86. Marik PE. Definition of sepsis: Not quite time to dump SIRS? Crit Care Med. 2002 March;30(3):706-8.

87. Liu S, Hou Y, Cui H. Clinical values of the early detection of serum procalcitonin, C-reactive protein and white blood cells for neonates with infectious diseases. Pak J Med Sci. 2016 Nov 15;32(6): 1326-9.

88. Prat C, Dominguez J, Rodrigo C, Giminez M, Azuara M, Jiminez O, et al. Elevated serum procalcitonin values correlate with renal scarring in children with urinary tract infection. Pediatric Infectious Disease Journal. 2003 May;22(5):438-42.

89. Chiesa C, Panero A, Rossi N, Stegagno M, de Giusti M, Osborn JF, et al. Reliability of Procalcitonin Concentrations for the Diagnosis of Sepsis in Critically Ill Neonates. Clinical Infectious Diseases. 1998 March;26(3):664-72.

90. Gervaix A, Pugin J. Usefulness of plasma procalcitonin determination in adults and children. Rev Med Suisse. 2005;1:872-7.

91. Smolkin V, Koren A, Raz R, Colodner R, Sakran W, Halevy R. Procalcitonin as a marker of acute pyelonephritis in infants and children. Pediatric Nephrology. 2002 June 8;17(6):409-12.

92. Benador N, Siegrist CA, Gendrel D, Greder C, Benador D, Assicot M, et al. Procalcitonin Is a Marker of Severity of Renal Lesions in Pyelonephritis. Pediatrics. 1998 Dec 1;102(6):1422-5.

93. Hirano T. Interleukin 6 and its Receptor: Ten Years Later. Int Rev Immunol. 1998 Jan 10;16(3-4):249-84.

94. Mathelier-Fusade P, Delers F, Engler R. Interleukin-8. Immunoanalysis & Specialized Biology. 1990 Dec;5(6):9-13.

95. Baggiolini M, Loetscher P, Moser B. Interleukin-8 and the chemokine family. Int J Immunopharmacol. 1995 Feb;17(2):103-8.

96. Roilides E, Papachristou F, Gioulekas E, Tsaparidou S, Karatzas N, Sotiriou J, et al. Increased Urine Interleukin-6 Concentrations Correlate with Pyelonephritic Changes on Tc-Dimercaptosuccinic Acid Scans in Neonates with Urinary Tract Infections. J Infect Dis. 1999 Sep;180(3):904-7.

97. Dunand O, Ulinski T, Bensman A. Urinary tract infections in children. EMC - Pediatrics - Infectious Diseases. 2008 Jan;3(3):1-7.

98. Clark CJ, Kennedy WA, Shortliffe LD. Urinary Tract Infection in Children: When to Worry. Urologic Clinics of North America. 2010 May 5;37(2):229-41.

99. Buettcher M, Trueck J, Niederer-Loher A, Heininger U, Agyeman P, Asner S, et al. Correction to: Swiss consensus recommendations on urinary tract infections in children. Eur J Pediatr. 2021 March 1;180(3):675-7.

100. Cochat P, Bacchetta J. Vesicoureteral reflux: the nephrologist's approach. Archives de Pédiatrie. 2009 June;16(6):909-11.

101. Mazzi S, Rohner K, Hayes W, Weitz M. Timing of voiding cystourethrography after febrile urinary tract infection in children: A systematic review. Vol. 105, Archives of Disease in Childhood. BMJ Publishing Group; 2020. p. 264-9.

102. Craig JC, Knight JF, Sureshkumar P, Lam A, Onikul E, Roy LP. Vesicoureteric reflux and timing of micturating cystourethrography after urinary tract infection. Arch Dis Child. 1997 March 1;76(3):275-7.

103. McDonald A, Scranton M, Gillespie R, Mahajan V, Edwards GA. Voiding Cystourethrograms and Urinary Tract Infections: How Long to Wait? Pediatrics. 2000 Apr 1;105(4):e50-e50.

104. Mahant S, To T, Friedman J. Timing of voiding cystourethrogram in the investigation of urinary tract infections in children. J Pediatr. 2001 Oct;139(4):568-71.

105. Condamin MC, Meyrier A. Contributions of current imaging to the diagnosis of acute pyelonephritis. Ultrasonography, computed tomography and scintigraphy. Med Mal Infect. 1991 Feb;21(2):89-95.

106. Millner R, Becknell B. Urinary tract infections. Pediatr Clin North Am. 2019 Feb;66(1):1-13.

107. Stein R, Dogan HS, Hoebeke P, Kocvara R, Nijman RJM, Radmayr C, et al. Urinary Tract Infections in Children: EAU/ESPU Guidelines. Eur Urol. 2015 March;67(3):546-58.

108. Bensman A. Acute pyelonephritis in children: What investigations? Journées Parisiennes de Pédiatrie. 2000;299-302.

109. Dunand O, Ulinski T, Bensman A. Urinary tract infections in children. EMC - Pediatrics - Infectious Diseases. 2008 Jan;3(3):1-7.

110. Stokland E, Hellstrom M, Jakobsson B, Sixt R. Imaging of renal scarring. Acta Paediatr. 2007 Jan 2;88:13-21.

111. Perli Goldraich N, Goldraich IH. Followup of Conservatively Treated Children with High and Low Grade Vesicoureteral Reflux: A Prospective Study. Journal of Urology. 1992 Nov;148(5):1688-92.

112. Pappas JN, Donnelly LF, Frush DP. Reduced Frequency of Sedation of Young Children with Multisection Helical CT. Radiology. 2000 June;215(3):897-9.

113. Borthne A, Nordshus T, Reiseter T, Geitung JT, Gjesdal KI, Babovic A, et al. MR urography: the future gold standard in paediatric urogenital imaging? Pediatr Radiol. 1999 August 23;29(9):694-701.

114. Nolte-Ernsting CC, Bücker A, Adam GB, Neuerburg JM, Jung P, Hunter DW, et al. Gadolinium-enhanced excretory MR urography after low-dose diuretic injection: comparison with conventional excretory urography. Radiology. 1998 Oct;209(1):147-57.

115. Kahloul N, Charfeddine L, Fatnassi R, Amri F. Malformative uropathies in children: about 71 cases. J Pediatr Pueric. 2010 juin;23(3):131-7.

116. Radet C, Champion G, Grimal I, Duverne C, Coupris L, Ginies JL, et al. Uropathies malformatives de diagnostic anténatal: prise en charge néonatale et devenir de 100 enfants nés entre 1988 et 1990 au CHU d'Angers. Archives de Pédiatrie. 1996 nov;3(11):1069-78.

117. Bouchaala F. Malformative uropathies in children: about 33 cases. Thèse de doctorat en médecine. Faculté de médecine de Sfax; 1983.

118. Mhiri R, Jlidi S, Khemakhem R, Boukadi A, ben Khalif A, Cadhi A, et al. Primary obstructive megaureter in children. À propos de 34 observations. Revue maghrébine de pédiatrie. 2001;11(6):299-305.

119. Ozel A, Alici Davutoglu E, Erenel H, Karsli MF, Korkmaz SO, Madazli R. Outcome after prenatal diagnosis of fetal urinary tract abnormalities: A tertiary center experience. Journal of the Turkish-German Gynecological Association. 2018 Apr 4;19(4):206-9.

120. Stocks A, Richards D, Frentzen B, Richard G. Correlation of Prenatal Renal Pelvic Anteroposterior Diameter with Outcome in Infancy. Journal of Urology. 1996;155(3):1050-2.

121. Nguyen HT, Benson CB, Bromley B, Campbell JB, Chow J, Coleman B, et al. Multidisciplinary consensus on the classification of prenatal

and postnatal urinary tract dilation (UTD classification system). J Pediatr Urol. 2014 Dec;10(6):982-98.

122. Tekgül S, Riedmiller H, Hoebeke P, Kocvara R, Nijman RJM, Radmayr C, et al. EAU Guidelines on Vesicoureteral Reflux in Children. Eur Urol. 2012 Sep;62(3):534-42.

123. Arlen AM, Cooper CS. Controversies in the Management of Vesicoureteral Reflux. Curr Urol Rep. 2015 Sep 22;16(9):64.

124. Hajiyev P, Burgu B. Contemporary Management of Vesicoureteral Reflux. Eur Urol Focus. 2017 Apr 1;3(2-3):181-8.

125. Michele Brophy M, Austin PF, Yan Y, Coplen DE. Vesicoureteral Reflux and Clinical Outcomes in Infants With Prenatally Detected Hydronephrosis. Journal of Urology. 2002 Oct;168(4 Part 2): 1716-9.

126. Phan V, Traubici J, Hershenfield B, Stephens D, Rosenblum ND, Geary DF. Vesicoureteral reflux in infants with isolated antenatal hydronephrosis. Pediatric Nephrology. 2003 Dec 1;18(12):1224-8.

127. Elder JS, Peters CA, Arant BS, Ewalt DH, Hawtrey CE, Hurwitz RS, et al. Pediatric Vesicoureteral Reflux Guidelines Panel Summary Report on the Management of Primary Vesicoureteral Reflux in Children. Journal of Urology. 1997 May;157(5):1846-51.

128. Williams G, Wei L, Lee A, Craig JC. Long-term antibiotics for preventing recurrent urinary tract infection in children. In: Williams G, editor. Cochrane Database of Systematic Reviews. Chichester, UK: John Wiley & Sons, Ltd; 2006.

129. Williams G, Craig JC. Prevention of recurrent urinary tract infection in children. Curr Opin Infect Dis. 2009 Feb;22(1):72-6.

130. Colen J, Docimo SG, Stanitski K, Sweeney DD, Wise B, Brandt P, et al. Dysfunctional elimination syndrome is a negative predictor for vesicoureteral reflux. J Pediatr Urol. 2006 Aug;2(4):312-5.

131. Greenfield SP. Antibiotic Prophylaxis in Pediatric Urology: An Update. Curr Urol Rep. 2011 Apr 13;12(2):126-31.

132. Greenfield SP, Chesney RW, Carpenter M, Moxey-Mims M, Nyberg L, Hoberman A, et al. Vesicoureteral Reflux: the RIVUR Study and the Way Forward. Journal of Urology. 2008 Feb;179(2):405-7.

133. Brandstrom P, Nevéus T, Sixt R, Stokland E, Jodal U, Hansson S. The Swedish Reflux Trial in Children: IV. Renal Damage. Journal of Urology. 2010 Jul;184(1):292-7.

134. Montini G, Rigon L, Zucchetta P, Fregonese F, Toffolo A, Gobber D, et al. Prophylaxis After First Febrile Urinary Tract Infection in Children? A Multicenter, Randomized, Controlled, Noninferiority Trial. Pediatrics. 2008 Nov 1;122(5):1064-71.

135. Pennesi M, Travan L, Peratoner L, Bordugo A, Cattaneo A, Ronfani L, et al. Is Antibiotic Prophylaxis in Children With Vesicoureteral Reflux Effective in Preventing Pyelonephritis and Renal Scars? A Randomized, Controlled Trial. Pediatrics. 2008 June 1;121(6):e1489-94.

136. Garin EH, Olavarria F, Nieto VG, Valenciano B, Campos A, Young L. Clinical Significance of Primary Vesicoureteral Reflux and Urinary Antibiotic Prophylaxis After Acute Pyelonephritis: A Multicenter, Randomized, Controlled Study. Pediatrics. 2006 March 1;117(3):626-32.

137. Brandstrom P, Esbjorner E, Herthelius M, Swerkersson S, Jodal U, Hansson S. The Swedish Reflux Trial in Children: III. Urinary Tract Infection Pattern. Journal of Urology. 2010 Jul;184(1):286-91.

138. Puri P, Granata C. Multicenter Survey of endoscopic treatment of vesicoureteral reflux using polytetrafluoroethylene. Journal of Urology. 1998 Sep;160(3):1007-11.

139. Steyaert H, Sattonnet C, Bloch C, Jaubert F, Galle P, Valla JS. Migration of PTFE paste particles to the kidney after treatment for vesico-ureteric reflux. BJU Int. 2000 Jan;85(1):168-9.

140. Lightner DJ. Review of the available urethral bulking agents. Curr Opin Urol. 2002 Jul;12(4):333-8.

141. Elder JS, Diaz M, Caldamone AA, Cendron M, Greenfield S, Hurwitz R, et al. Endoscopic Therapy for Vesicoureteral Reflux: A Meta-Analysis. I. Reflux Resolution and Urinary Tract Infection. Journal of Urology. 2006 Feb;175(2):716-22.

142. Holmdahl G, Brandstrom P, Lackgren G, Sillén U, Stokland E, Jodal U, et al. The Swedish Reflux Trial in Children: II. Vesicoureteral Reflux Outcome. Journal of Urology. 2010 Jul;184(1):280-5.

143. Merrot T, Ouedraogo I, Hery Géraldine, Alessandrini P. Preliminary results: endoscopic treatment of vesicoureteral reflux in children: prospective comparative study Deflux®/Coaptite®. Progrés en Urologie. 2005;15:1114-9.

144. Carpentier PJ, Bettink PJ, Hop WCJ, Schroder FH. Reflux-A Retrospective Study of 100 Ureteric Reimplantations by the Politano-Leadbetter Method and 100 by the Cohen Technique. Journal of Urology. 1983 Apr;129(4):889-889.

145. Sillén U. Vesicoureteral reflux in infants. Pediatric Nephrology. 1999 May 19;13(4):355-61.

146. Peycelon M, Audry G. The role of surgery in the management of reflux.
vesico-ureteral disease in children. Archives of Pediatrics. 2009 Dec;16(12):1598-602.

147. Tanagho EA. Surgical Revision of the incompetennt ureterovesical junction: A critical analysis of techniques and requirements. Br J Urol. 1970 Aug;42(4):410-24.

148. Cortesse A, Cariou C. Nephro-ureterectomy. EMC Techniques chirurgicales - Urologie. 2002;41-120.

149. Schanstra J, Bascands JL. Pathophysiology of obstructive uropathies: contribution of genetically modified animals. Archives of Pediatrics. 2003 Oct;10(10):903-10.

150. Gohimont N, Muteganya R, Tondeur M. Role of radio-isotopic functional imaging in the work-up of pyelo-ureteral junction syndrome

in children. Rev Med Brux. 2020 Feb 1;41(1):10-8.

151. Choi YH, Cheon JE, Kim WS, Kim IO. Ultrasonography of hydronephrosis in the newborn: a practical review. Ultrasonography. 2016 Jul 1;35(3):198-211.

152. Menon P, Rao KLN, Sodhi KS, Bhattacharya A, Saxena AK, Mittal BR. Hydronephrosis: Comparison of extrinsic vessel versus intrinsic ureteropelvic junction obstruction groups and a plea against the vascular hitch procedure. J Pediatr Urol. 2015 Apr;11(2):80.e1-80.e6.

153. Audry G, de Vries P, Bonnard A. Particularities of the treatment of pyeloureteral junction anomaly in children. Ann Urol (Paris). 2006 Feb;40(1):28-38.

154. Hyh Rantomalala M, Rabarijaona A, Rakotoarisoa B, Razafindramboa H, Radesa FS. Ureteral transposition to treat pyeloureteral junction syndrome by crossing the inferior polar pedicle: About two cases. Med Afr Noire. 2003;50(8-9):377-9.

155. Buisson P, Ricard J, Boudailliez B, Canarelli JP. Evolution of the management of pyeloureteral junction syndrome. Archives de Pédiatrie. 2003 March;10(3):215-20.

156. Amadou I, Coulibaly Y, Coulibaly O, Keita M, Coulibaly M, Coulibaly Y, et al. Syndrome de la Jonction Pyélo-Urétérale: Aspects Cliniques et Thérapeutiques au CHU Gabriel Toure. Health Sciences and Disease. 2018;19(3):69-72.

157. Tlemsani Maghraoui Z. Pyeloureteral junction syndrome (à-propos de 38 cas). Thesis for doctorate in medicine. Faculty of Medicine and Pharmacy, Rabat; 2021.

158. Descotes JL. Treatment of adult pyeloureteral junction stenosis. Progrès en Urologie. 2013 Nov;23(14):1172-6.

159. Harrow BR, Bagrodia A, Olweny EO, Faddegon S, Cadeddu JA, Gahan JC. Renal Function After Laparoendoscopic Single Site Pyeloplasty. Journal of Urology. 2013 Aug;190(2):565-9.

160. Diakité ML, Coulibaly Y, Berthé HJG, Merrot T, Chaumoitre K,

Alessandrini P, et al. Primary obstructive megaureter: therapeutic strategies about 30 cases. African Journal of Urology. 2013 June;19(2):107-12.

161. WILLIAMS DI, HULME-MOIR I. PRIMARY OBSTRUCTIVE MEGAURETER. Br J Urol. 1970 Apr;42(2): 140-9.

162. Brown T, Mandell J, Lebowitz R. Neonatal hydronephrosis in the era of sonography. American Journal of Roentgenology. 1987 May 1;148(5):959-63.

163. Ghanmi S, ben Hamouda H, Krichene I, Soua H, Ayadi A, Souissi MM, et al. Management and evolution of primary mega-ureters of antenatal discovery. Progrès en Urologie. 2011 Jul;21(7):486-91.

164. Chertin B, Pollack A, Koulikov D, Rabinowitz R, Shen O, Hain D, et al. Long-term follow up of antenatally diagnosed megaureters. J Pediatr Urol. 2008 June;4(3):188-91.

165. Stamilio DM, Morgan MA. DIAGNOSIS OF FETAL RENAL ANOMALIES. Obstet Gynecol Clin North Am. 1998 Sept;25(3):527-52.

166. Gargah T, Gharbi Y, ben Moussa M, Kaabar N, Lakhoua MR. Valves de L'urethètre Postérieur. A Propos de 44 Cas. Tunis Med. 2010;88(08):557-62.

167. Perks AE, MacNeily AE, Blair GK. Posterior urethral valves. J Pediatr Surg. 2002 Jul;37(7):1105-7.

168. Papillard S, Grapin C, Montagne JP. Urinary tract dilatation identified in the antenatal period: conduct of postnatal diagnosis. Archives de Pédiatrie. 2006 March;13(3):299-301.

169. Allouch G. Antenatal screening uropathies: 4 years of experience, 147 patients. J Urol (Paris). 1993;99(1):11-5.

170. Khemakhem R, ben Ahmed Y, Mefteh S, Jlidi S, Charieg A, Louati H, et al. Valves of the posterior urethra: about 38 cases. J Pediatr Pueric. 2012 Oct;25(5):242-8.

171. Traisman ES. Clinical Management of Urinary Tract Infections. Pediatr Ann. 2016 Apr;45(4):e108-11.

172. Balighian E, Burke M. Urinary Tract Infections in Children. Pediatr Rev. 2018 Jan 1;39(1):3-12.

173. Schlager TA. Urinary Tract Infections in Infants and Children. Mulvey MA, Stapleton AE, Klumpp DJ, editors. Microbiol Spectr. 2016 Oct;4(5):69-77.

174. Buxeraud J, Faure S. Cephalosporins. Actualités Pharmaceutiques. 2021 June;60(607):S24-7.

175. Gaudelus J. Antibiotic therapy of acute pyelonephritis: which treatment to propose? Archives de Pédiatrie. 1999 Jan;6(2):S403-5.

176. Cohen R, Raymond J, Faye A, Gillet Y, Grimprel E. Prise en charge des infections urinaires de l'enfant. Recommandations du groupe de pathologie infectieuse pédiatrique de la Société française de pédiatrie et de la Société de pathologie infectieuse de langue française. Archives de Pédiatrie. 2015 June;22(6):665-71.

177. Delbet JD, Lorrot M, Ulinski T. An update on new antibiotic prophylaxis and treatment for urinary tract infections in children. Expert Opin Pharmacother. 2017 Oct 13;18(15):1619-25.

178. Cohen R, Raymond J, Launay E, Gillet Y, Minodier P, Dubos F, et al. Antimicrobial treatment of urinary tract infections in children. Archives de Pédiatrie. 2017 Dec;24(12):S22-5.

179. Magin EC, Garcia-Garcia JJ, Sert SZ, Giralt AG, Cubells CL. Efficacy of Short-Term Intravenous Antibiotic in Neonates With Urinary Tract Infection. Pediatr Emerg Care. 2007 Feb;23(2):83-6.

180. Nathanson S, Deschênes G. Urinary antibiotic prophylaxis. Archives de Pédiatrie. 2002 May;9(5):511-8.

181. Beetz R, Bachmann H, Gatermann S, Keller H, Kuwertz-Broking E, Misselwitz J, et al. Urinary tract infections in infancy and childhood: consensus recommendations for diagnosis, therapy and prophylaxis. Urologe. 2007 Feb;46(2):112-23.

182. The management of urinary tract infection in children. Drug Ther Bull. 1997 Sept 1;35(9):65-9.

183. Simforoosh N, Tabibi A, Khalili SAR, Soltani MH, Afjehi A, Aalami F, et al. Neonatal circumcision reduces the incidence of asymptomatic urinary tract infection: A large prospective study with long-term follow up using Plastibell. J Pediatr Urol. 2012 June;8(3):320-3.

184. Sorokan ST, Finlay JC, Jefferies AL. Neonatal circumcision. Paediatr Child Health. 2015 August 1;20(6):316-20.

185. Oreskovic NM, Sembrano EU. Repeat Urine Cultures in Children Who Are Admitted With Urinary Tract Infections. Pediatrics. 2007 Feb 1;119(2):e325-9.

186. Currie ML, Mitz L, Raasch CS, Greenbaum LA. Follow-up Urine Cultures and Fever in Children With Urinary Tract Infection. Arch Pediatr Adolesc Med. 2003 Dec 1;157(12):1237-40.

187. Ajrafi M. Infection urinaire febriles de l'enfant du diagnostic à la prise en charge. Thesis for doctorate in medicine. Faculty of Medicine and Pharmacy Rabat; 2022.

188. Heffner VA, Gorelick MH. Pediatric Urinary Tract Infection. Clin Pediatr Emerg Med. 2008 Dec;9(4):233-7.

189. Anoukoum T, Agbodjan-Djossou O, Atakouma YD, Bakonde B, Folligan K, Boukari B, et al. Epidemiological and etiological aspects of childhood urinary tract infection in the pediatric department of CHU-Campus de Lomé (Togo). Ann Urol (Paris). 2001;35(3):178-84.

190. Sinha MD, Postlethwaite RJ. Urinary tract infections and the long-term risk of hypertension. Current Paediatrics. 2003 Dec;13(7):508-12.

191. Sedberry-Ross S, Pohl HG. Urinary tract infections in children. Curr Urol Rep. 2008 March 9;9(2):165-71.

192. Smyth AR, Judd BA. Compliance with antibiotic prophylaxis in urinary tract infection. Arch Dis Child. 1993 Feb 1;68(2):235-6.

193. Faust WC, Diaz M, Pohl HG. Incidence of Post-Pyelonephritic Renal

Scarring: A Meta-Analysis of the Dimercapto-Succinic Acid Literature. Journal of Urology. 2009 Jan;181(1):290-8.

194. Jakobsson B, Berg U, Svensson L. Renal scarring after acute pyelonephritis. Arch Dis Child. 1994 Feb 1;70(2):111-5.

SUMMARY

Neonatal urinary tract infection (NUTI) is a unique entity, characterized by an unspecific, often misleading clinical symptomatology and frequent association with malformative uropathy. Neonatal UTI is a pathology that requires prompt medical attention because of its potential to lead to severe complications. Early recognition of symptoms, accurate diagnosis and appropriate treatment are essential to preserve the renal and general health of the newborn. Prevention through good hygiene and monitoring of at-risk newborns also helps to reduce the incidence of this infection. In short, a proactive and systematic approach is crucial to ensure the well-being of the youngest patients.

Conclusion: Urinary tract infection remains a worrying pathology in newborns. Knowing how to prevent it and treat it in time can reduce morbidity and mortality.

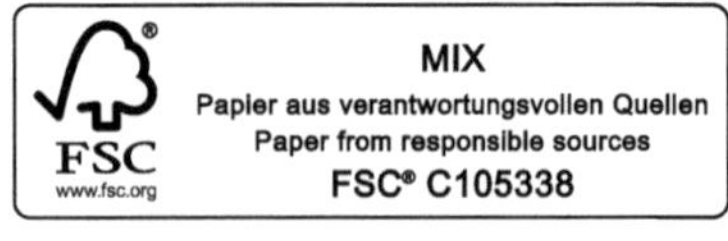

Printed by Books on Demand GmbH, Norderstedt / Germany